REMEMBERING THE FRONTIER

OUR HORSEBACK HERITAGE

AMY PENNINGTON BRUDNICKI

BRUDNICKI-PENN PUBLISHING

About the Covers:

Front Cover: This striking photo is one of Mary Breckinridge in her later years. Photo used with permission from Frontier Nursing University.

Back Cover: This serene photo is one I took in Mary Breckinridge's bedroom in the Big House on a crisp, thirty-two degree October morning.

Copyright © 2020 by Amy Pennington Brudnicki

All rights reserved.

No part of this book may be reproduced in any form or by any electronic or mechanical means, including information storage and retrieval systems, without written permission from the author, except for the use of brief quotations in a book review.

DEDICATION

Dedicated to the people of Leslie County and FNS babies everywhere.

Leslie County is deep-rooted in the legacy of Mary Breckinridge and the Frontier Nursing Service. Let's make it our mission to pass along stories to future generations who will never experience her work firsthand, but who wouldn't be here if not for her.

Our heritage is something to be proud of. Let's be purposeful in assuring that our history is never forgotten . . .

~ Amy Pennington Brudnicki
FNS Baby

CONTENTS

Introduction	xi
Frontier Memories	xii
Excerpt	xiv
Jutting Rocks on Wendover	xv
1. Mary Breckinridge	1
2. Things to Consider . . .	3
3. Memories	4
4. The Saddlebag Baby	5
5. FNS Babies & Their Midwives	6
6. FNS Babies	7
7. Layette Bundles	8
8. Special Nurse-Midwives & Couriers	9
9. Creek Clinics	10
10. Outpost Nursing Centers	11
11. Baby Bill	12
12. Wendover Structures	13
13. Legendary Stone Steps	14
14. Acts of Service	15
15. Those Wide Neighborhoods	16
16. Frontier Nursing Service Occupations	17
17. Transportation	18
18. The Big House Memories	19
19. Animals	20
20. Cornerstone	21
21. Mary Breckinridge	22
22. Saddlebags	27
23. FNS Uniforms	28
24. THE OLD HYDEN HOSPITAL Dedication: June 26, 1928	30
25. Then vs Now	33
26. FNS Properties	35

27. The Mary Breckinridge Festival	37
28. Naming of Wendover	39
29. THE BIG HOUSE Wendover	40
30. "DEDICATION OF LIGHTS" The Big House	43
31. THE GARDEN HOUSE Wendover	45
32. THE GARDEN HOUSE Wendover	47
ST. CHRISTOPHER'S CHAPEL Hospital Hill	49
33. ST. CHRISTOPHER'S CHAPEL Hospital Hill	51
34. The Upper Shelf	54
35. MARY BRECKINRIDGE HOSPITAL Dedication: January 5, 1975	56
36. Old Christmas	58
37. FNS Quarterly Bulletins	59
38. Special FNS Horses	60
39. "THE NIGHT BEFORE CHRISTMAS" By Betty Palethorp, R.N., S.C.M.	62
40. "REFLECTIONS" By Goldie Davidson	64
41. Heritage	68
42. Preserving History	70
The Big House	71
43. Mary Breckinridge's Canes & Walking Sticks	72
44. Beautiful China	74
45. CHRISTMAS PLAY 1975	75
46. Fifth Generation Maggard	76
47. Days Gone By	77
48. "A CURB BIT HANGS SILENTLY, Quote by Audrey Maggard Clowers	78
49. THE UPPER SHELF Photo Taken 2010	79

50. VINTAGE BOOKS & BOOKCASES The Big House Living Room	80
51. BOOK SIGNING September 21, 2019	81
52. Mardi Cottage	82
53. Haggin Nurses Dorm	83
54. STONE STEPS Photo Taken 2018	84
55. Following in the Steps of Mary Breckinridge,	85
56. STONE STEPS October 2015	86
57. WENDOVER October 17, 2020	87
58. Rock Wall	88
59. Picturesque Grounds	89
60. THE BIG HOUSE December 2017	90
61. RIVERBANK 10/17/2020	91
62. ROCKY RIVERBED 10/18/2015	92
63. ST. CHRISTOPHER'S CHAPEL Hospital HIll	93
64. St. Christopher's Chapel	94
65. VINTAGE BOOKS Hospital Hill	95
66. ORGAN Hospital Hill	96
67. CHRISTMAS PLAY 1975	97
68. ENCLOSED PORCH December 14, 2018	98
69. WENDOVER CHRISTMAS PLAY 1975	99
70. THE DOG TROT DINING ROOM Photo Taken December 14, 2018	100

71. THE FRONT DINING ROOM   101
    12/14/2018

72. THE FRONT ROOM   102
    December 14, 2018

73. NATIVITY PLAY   103
    1975

74. CHRISTMAS TREE IN THE LIVING ROOM OF   104
    THE BIG HOUSE
    Photo by Amy Pennington Brudnicki

75. BEAUTIFUL FIREPLACE   106
    Photo taken December 2017

76. STAIRCASE   107
    December 27, 2019

77. LIVING ROOM WINDOW   108
    Hillside Overlooking the Middle Fork River

78. THE DOG TROT DINING ROOM   109
    October 2015

79. WENDOVER NATIVITY PLAY   110
    1975

80. THE MANGER   111
    October 17, 2015

81. Exposed Beam Ceiling   112

82. VINTAGE BOOKCASE IN MARY BRECKINRIDGE'S   113
    BEDROOM
    October 17, 2015

83. CONTINUING THE TRADITION   114
    Hurricane Creek Cousins

84. WENDOVER CHRISTMAS PLAY   115
    1975

85. LITTLE ANGELS   116
    Tina McKinney, Michelle Cornett, and Amy Maggard

86. Explorers   118

87. Young Explorers   119

88. AMY PENNINGTON BRUDNICKI   120
    Legendary Florence Nightingale Brick from her home. It is
    said that rubbing the brick brings good luck.

89. VINTAGE BOOKS October 17, 2015	121
90. LUNCH WITH FRIENDS December 2019	122
91. Vintage FNS Photos	123
92. MARY BRECKINRIDGE The Frontier Nursing Service	124
93. Frontier Nursing Service	125
94. THE BIG HOUSE & Helen Browne	126
95. The Old Hyden Hospital	127
96. Christmas Dinner with the Couriers, 1928	128
97. Mary Breckinridge	129
98. The Original Garden House	130
99. The Original Garden House	131
100. TRANSPORTATION, OLD VS. NEW Betty Lester in Jeep	132
101. BETTY LESTER Hospital Hill	133
102. The Wendover Cabin	134
103. The Saddlebag Baby	135
104. FNS Nurses	136
105. Mary Breckinridge	137
106. Mary Breckinridge	138
107. Couriers Washing the Jeep	139
108. Mary Breckinridge	140
109. The Wendover Barn	141
110. HOME DELIVERY The walls are covered with newspaper, something that was common in mountain homes.	142
111. Days Gone By	143
112. Couriers on Horseback	144
113. Courier in Jeep	145
114. The Original Wendover Barn	146
115. Christmas Nativity Play	147
116. The Wendover Cabin	148
117. Log Cabin Chapel	149
118. Pig Alley	150

119.	Nurses on Horseback	151
120.	A Young Mary Breckinridge	152
121.	Quarterly Bulletin Photos	153
122.	FIRST QUARTERLY BULLETIN The Kentucky Committee for Mothers and Babies, Predecessor to FNS	154
123.	CHILDREN'S OUTDOOR WARD The Quarterly Bulletin of the Frontier Nursing Service, Inc.	155
124.	FLOATING LOGS DOWN THE MIDDLE FORK The Quarterly Bulletin of the Frontier Nursing Service, Inc.	156
125.	BUILDING THE CHAPEL St. Christopher's Chapel	157
126.	CHAPEL CONSTRUCTION Photo by Mr. J.A. Riordan	158
127.	Molly Lee	159
128.	ANNA MAY JANUARY Beloved Nurse-Midwife	160
129.	CHRISTMAS PAGEANT Photo by Anne Cundle	161
130.	A BABY A DAY Spring 1931 FNS Quarterly Bulletin (14I & 14J)	162
131.	WENDOVER GEESE Photo by Hought Barber	165
132.	HELEN BROWNE & ROGERS BEASLEY Photo by Gabrielle Beasley	166
133.	COURIER MARGO SQUIBB AS SANTA AND JACK BEGLEY Photo by Gabrielle Beasley	167
134.	Frontier Nurses	168
135.	CREEK CLINIC Photo by Toad Hall	169
136.	MARLENE WOOTON Ten Thousandth FNS Baby	170
137.	STEPS TO OLD HYDEN HOSPITAL Photo by Toad Hall	171
138.	Wee Stone House	172
139.	The Upper Shelf	173

140. Party at the Upper Shelf — 174
141. MARY FRANCES MORGAN — 175
    Wendover Christmas Play
142. EARLY DAYS — 176
    Living Room of The Big House
143. Mountain Home Visit — 177
144. Kate Ireland — 178
145. MARY BRECKINRIDGE HOSPITAL — 179
    Photo by Rufus Fugate
146. CORNERSTONE CONTENTS — 180
    Photos by Gabrielle Beasley
147. CHASTITY LYNN DEBORD — 182
    First Baby Born in the New Mary Breckinridge Hospital
148. SAYINGS OF OUR CHILDREN — 183
    Quote by Tina McKinney
149. MOUNTAIN SCHOOLHOUSE — 184
    Artist Unknown
150. GLORIA NAPIER — 185
    Littlest Angel
151. COAL COUNTRY GRASS — 186
    Local Musicians Donate Proceeds to the Leslie County Volunteer Fire Department
152. NATIVITY PLAY — 187
    At Wendover Garden House
153. CHRISTMAS PLAY — 188
    At Wendover Garden House
154. GRETCHEN SHEPHERD — 189
    Centennial Princess
155. Betty Lester — 190
156. CHRISTMAS NATIVITY PLAY — 191
    Re-enactment by Local Children
157. NATIVITY PAGEANT ANGELS — 192
    Wendover
158. CHRISTMAS NATIVITY PAGEANT SHEPHERDS AND WISEMEN — 194
    Wendover
159. Gratitude — 196

160. Acknowledgements	198
161. References	204
162. References	205
About the Author	211
Also by Amy Pennington Brudnicki	212

INTRODUCTION

Could one dollar possibly change your life? How about something that was absolutely free?

The answer may surprise you...

FRONTIER MEMORIES

This serene photo is one I took in Mary Breckinridge's bedroom in the Big House on a crisp, thirty-two degree October morning.

It was my first time staying at the Wendover Bed & Breakfast, but it certainly wouldn't be my last.

That first morning, after gazing upon the photo, I knew in my heart that it would be special—I just didn't know to what extent.

Five years later, that reason became apparent to me when I chose this as the back cover of an important book of Leslie County history. I see this as Mary Breckinridge's story floating out, memory by memory...

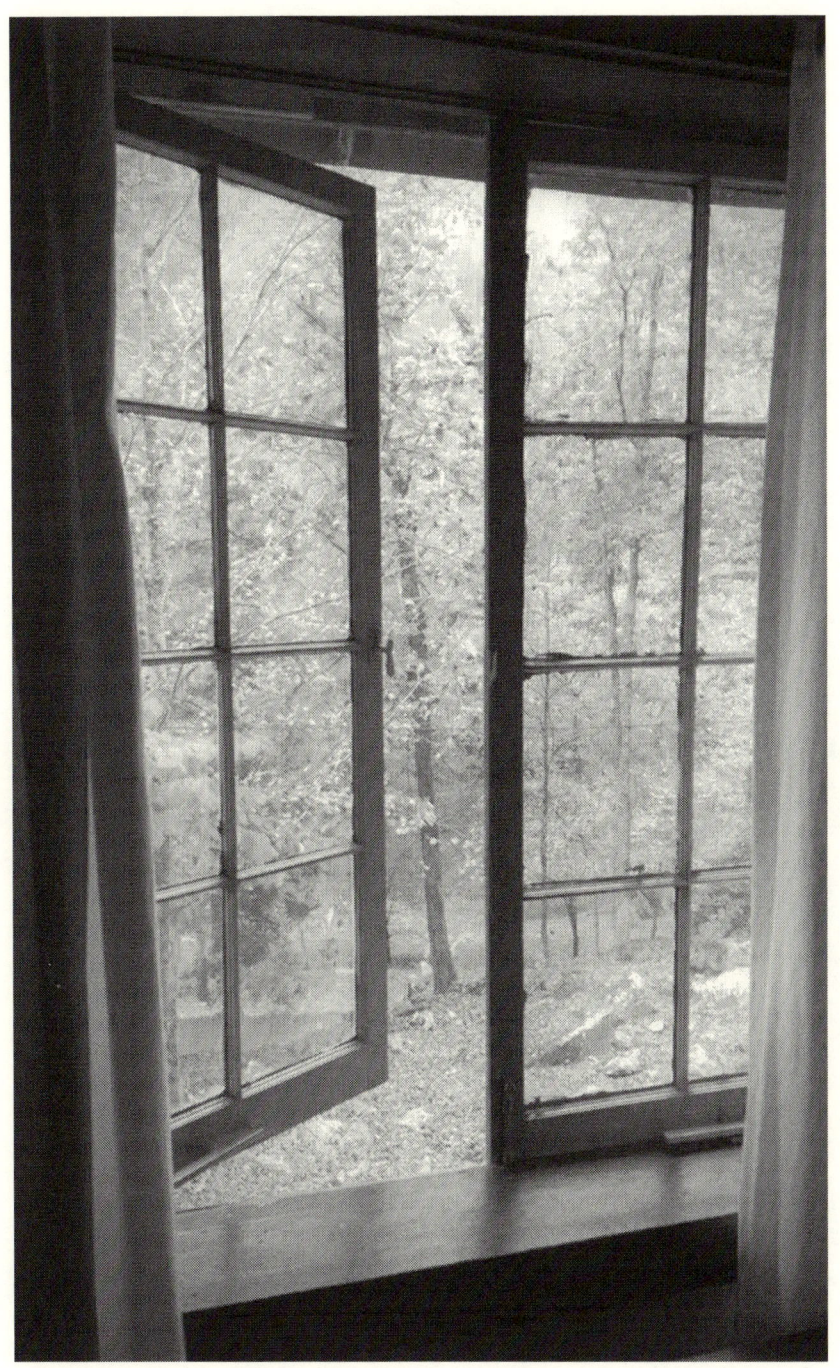

EXCERPT
WIDE NEIGHBORHOODS

"It was one of my rides alone that I first saw Wendover. Of course it wasn't Wendover then, but I knew it would be. It was purely by accident that I happened to be riding along the Middle Fork of the Kentucky River. I was on my way to Stinnett and Beech Fork where the direct road lay up Muncy Creek and across a gap to Stinnett Creek. A dear girl, Pauline Brashear, whom I had met at the Buyers' dormitory in Hyden, begged me to turn off at Muncy Creek and follow a detour of some miles along the river that would take me past the home of some of her people. She went ahead of me to tell them I would be there for the noon dinner. So the first of many thousands of times, I rode down Muncy Creek, forded the Middle Fork and rode slowly along its banks. I thought I had never seen anything lovelier than the lay of the land with its southern exposure facing the great North Mountain. When I raised my eyes to towering forest trees, and then let them fall on a cleared place where one might have a garden, when I passed some jutting rocks, I fell in love. To myself and to my horse I said, 'Someday I'm going to build me a log house right there.' Two years later I did." (4)

— MARY BRECKINRIDGE

JUTTING ROCKS ON WENDOVER
AS STRIKING TODAY AS THEY WERE A HUNDRED YEARS AGO WHEN MARY BRECKINRIDGE FIRST SAW THEM

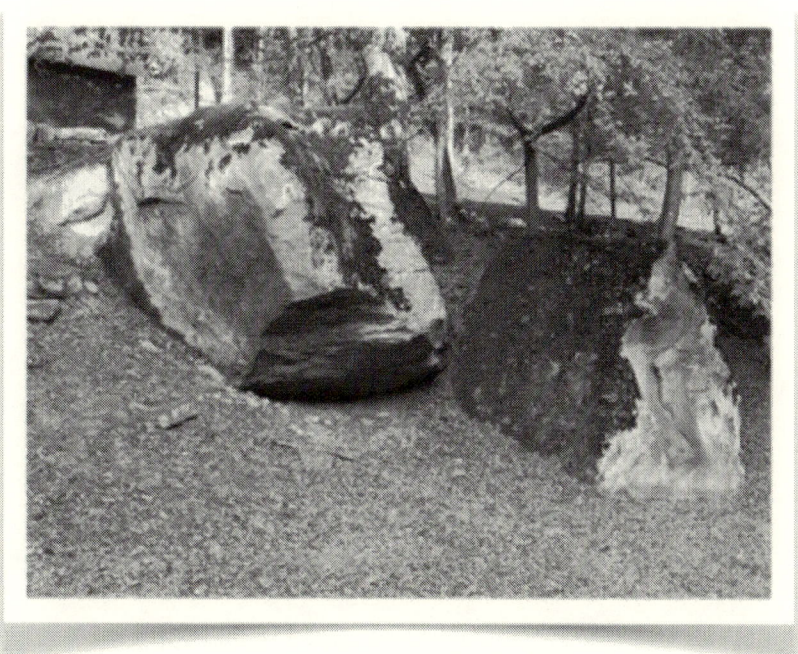

Photo by Amy Pennington Brudnicki

1

MARY BRECKINRIDGE

IN 1925, Mary Carson Breckinridge established The Kentucky Committee for Mothers and Babies. In 1928, the name was changed to the Frontier Nursing Service—or, FNS, for short—a program that brought healthcare to families in the rugged terrain of rural eastern Kentucky. [A]

Traveling by horseback, Mary Breckinridge and her team of midwives provided quality healthcare to mothers and babies, drastically improving the infant-mortality rate in the Appalachian Mountains.

Being that nurses and midwives had to carry all their supplies with them when they assisted in home births, the saddlebags on the horses were always full of equipment and seemingly always bulging. [B][C]

Because of this, mountain children in Leslie County thought the saddlebags were full of babies, and so the term, Saddlebag Babies, was born. [B][C]

. . .

HAVING LOST two young children of her own, helping these families became Mary Breckinridge's life mission.

SHE DID SO MUCH MORE than birth babies, though. She formed lasting relationships with the citizens of our tight-knit community of Hyden, Kentucky.

She facilitated community outreach programs through her remote Creek Clinics and Outpost Nursing Centers. She hosted community holiday gatherings at her beloved Wendover, the location of her two-story log cabin, The Big House, and she would go on to oversee the construction of Hyden's first hospital, the old Hyden Hospital on Hospital Hill, completed in 1928. [B)(C)(A)(3)]

In addition to FNS, the hospital, and the outpost nursing centers that she sat up throughout the county, Mary Breckinridge had the foresight to see that nurses were trained to become nurse-midwives.

In 1939, she created the Frontier School of Midwifery and Family Nursing. [A]

MARY BRECKINRIDGE HAD a giving spirit and a heart of love. Of all the places in the world she could've gone, of the places she could have chosen to live and work, she chose us and our Appalachian Mountains.

WALK with me back in time as we remember the wonderful legacy of Mary Breckinridge—as we assure the Frontier is never forgotten...

2

THINGS TO CONSIDER...

ON THE FOLLOWING PAGES, you'll see how Mary Breckinridge came to Leslie County nearly one hundred years ago and forever changed lives in the rural, Eastern Kentucky community.

This keepsake book of Frontier history begins with questions to consider and discuss with your loved ones.

Mary Breckinridge history, FNS history, and vintage photos complete this collection.

3

MEMORIES

Do you have personal memories of Mary Breckinridge? If not, do you remember your family sharing stories about her and the Frontier Nursing Service?

4

THE SADDLEBAG BABY

Were you a Saddlebag Baby? If not, was anyone in your family a Saddlebag Baby?

The saddlebag baby has direct knowledge of the Frontier Nursing Service. This is one of the greatest generations for so many reasons.

5

FNS BABIES & THEIR MIDWIVES

Do you know any details surrounding your birth? For example, were you born at home, or were you born in the hospital? Do you know the name of the nurse-midwife who delivered you?

6

FNS BABIES

Can you list the FNS babies in your family? If you and your loved ones are from Leslie County, I imagine that'll be a rather impressive list.

7

LAYETTE BUNDLES

EVERY NEW MOTHER who had a baby at the old Hyden Hospital was sent home with layette bundles. Some items included in the bundles were: receiving blankets, baby gowns, cloth diapers, diaper pins, soap, and a variety of other items . . .

Do you remember any other items from your own child's bundle?
    Do you still have any of those items? [B]

SPECIAL NURSE-MIDWIVES & COURIERS

Miss Anna May January was a special nurse-midwife to my family, having visited three generations of my family. Molly Lee and Sharon Koser were also special to us. [B]

Do you remember the special nurse-midwives or couriers who visited your own family?

9

CREEK CLINICS

DID the nurses ever come to a single household in your neighborhood or holler to provide immunizations for many families at one time? They referred to these visits as *Creek Clinics*. Do you remember whose house they came to, and who all was there? [B][C]

10

OUTPOST NURSING CENTERS

IN ADDITION to the old Hyden Hospital, Mary Breckinridge saw to it that remote outpost nursing centers were set up throughout the county. Clinics included Beech Fork Center, Big Creek Center, Wendover Outpost Center, the Wooton Clinic, and many others. If you sought service beyond the hospital, which outpost clinic did you go to? [A][B][3]

11

BABY BILL

If you had a Saddlebag Baby or had a baby in the hospital, do you remember how much your baby bill was?

Through oral history, I've discovered that bills were sometimes settled in manners that stretched beyond the dollar. Goods and services were also accepted. Do you have any examples of this?

12

WENDOVER STRUCTURES

Do you remember the Wendover Cabin—also referred to as the Log Chapel—or the Upper Shelf and Lower Shelf Cabins that used to stand on Wendover? [A][2]

Did you ever go inside them? Can you describe them?

LEGENDARY STONE STEPS

Do you recall the stone steps up to the old Hyden Hospital?

Did you ever climb them?

14

ACTS OF SERVICE

BECAUSE OF MARY BRECKINRIDGE and her spirit of giving, did you, or someone you know, become a nurse or healthcare worker?

15

THOSE WIDE NEIGHBORHOODS

MARY BRECKINRIDGE WROTE a book called Wide Neighborhoods. If you haven't read it, get a copy. She was a good human, and we'd each benefit from her lead. If you have read Wide Neighborhoods, what were some interesting or noteworthy things you read about?

16

FRONTIER NURSING SERVICE OCCUPATIONS

Have you, or anyone you know, worked at Wendover or Hospital Hill for FNS?

What jobs were done there?

TRANSPORTATION

IN THE EARLY days of FNS, transportation was almost exclusively achieved by horseback. In later years, Jeeps were phased in as the primary means of transportation.

THEY HAD names for both the horses and the Jeeps. Do you remember any of the names? [A]

18

THE BIG HOUSE MEMORIES

Did you ever spend some time at the Wendover Big House—either, when it was a residence or as a guest at the Bed & Breakfast?

Did you ever stay overnight or eat a meal there? (A)

19

ANIMALS

Wendover has always been well known for its love of animals.
   The grounds have been home to many horses, dogs, pigs, cows, chickens, geese . . . [B][C][3]

Can you think of any memorable Wendover animals?

Do you remember their names?

20

CORNERSTONE
MARY BRECKINRIDGE HOSPITAL

In 1970, a ground-breaking ceremony was held for the new hospital, The Mary Breckinridge Hospital.

In 1975, the building was completed.

The cornerstone of the hospital includes special items.
  Do you know what they are? [3W]

21

MARY BRECKINRIDGE
HISTORY

- Mary Carson Breckinridge was born in Memphis, Tennessee, February 17, 1881. [5]
- Mother of two—Polly, who lived only a few hours, and Breckie, who passed away when he was four-years-old [A]
- Born into a family of privilege, one that could have afforded her any dream she dared to dream, Mary Breckinridge would go on to become a public health servant and advocate for mothers, babies, and families in one of the poorest regions in the country.
- Began her work in Leslie County at the age of 44
- Established the Committee for Mothers and Babies, 1925 [A]
- Founded the Frontier Nursing Service, 1928 [A]
- Responsible for Hyden's First Hospital, Hyden Hospital, 1928 [C]
- Began the Frontier School of Midwifery and Family Nursing, 1939 [A]
- World Traveler [4]

- Bi-lingual, even teaching French at one time [5]
- Educated in the United States and Abroad [5]
- Writer and Published Author
- Animal Lover
- Kind, Compassionate Soul
- Lover of Leslie County
- Neighbor
- Earth Angel to all of Leslie County

A MOUNTAIN GRANNY

ANYONE WHO KNOWS the history of Mary Breckinridge knows that her reach went beyond birthing babies.

Sure, that's what she was initially known for, and that's a tremendous legacy. But, once she settled on Wendover, she became a friend and neighbor to many, mentoring, teaching, encouraging . . . a mountain granny, of sorts.

In the 1940s, my Aunt Audrey was a young girl. It was Christmastime, and she would soon be introduced to the Christmas Nativity plays at Wendover.

She shared a sweet story with me about Mary Breckinridge.

Aunt Audrey said she was a shy little girl. When it came time to say her part in the play, she got scared and forgot the words.

As any great encourager would do, Aunt Audrey said that Mary Breckinridge sat behind her during the play and whispered the words she was to say when it was time to say them.

She spoke of Mary Breckinridge so adoringly. I'm accustomed to hearing about Mary Breckinridge from the perspective of an adult. But because Aunt Audrey shared her story, I saw Mary Breckinridge through the eyes of a child. And that was a special moment.

. . .

AUNT AUDREY WENT on to share another story about, what she called, "The Mountain Grapevine."

Where she lived, the river separated her home and Wendover.

She said that her mother, Callie, was out walking one day when a vicious dog lunged at her and attacked her.

On the other side of the mountain, unbeknownst to her mother, a hunter was in the mountains and saw what happened.

Being that he could reach The Big House faster than he could cross the river, he ran down to Wendover and told them what happened.

Aunt Audrey said that, by the time her mother had limped home, the FNS nurses had beat her there. Mrs. Breckinridge had sent them.

She went on to say that Mary Breckinridge saved her mother's life because she insisted on diagnostic testing. As it turned out, the dog was rabid.

Mary Breckinridge provided treatments for Mrs. Morgan, saving her life.

Years later, Mrs. Morgan would go on to care for Mrs. Breckinridge, as many did, in her final years.

"THE TRUMPETS SOUNDED"

The Spring 1965 Quarterly Bulletin features Mary Breckinridge on the cover. Sitting high atop a dark horse, she's clothed in the legendary blue summer nurses' uniform. [3A]

In life, she seemingly shied away from the focus of the spotlight, choosing, instead, to showcase the success of her mission and the work of her nurse-midwives.

However, it's fitting that her photo graced *this* special issue. All the quarterly bulletins were special in that they were filled with wonderful and interesting tidbits. But, this issue was increasingly special because it was the last one she would ever work on, having worked on it until one day prior to her death.

On May 16, 1965, Mary Breckinridge passed away in her bedroom of The Big House.

In the Spring 1965 edition of the Quarterly Bulletin, Betty Lester writes a poignant article titled, *"The Trumpets Sounded."* It's a detailed account of Mary Breckinridge's final hours, as well as noteworthy events surrounding her funeral. [3A]

FNS Quarterly Bulletin Spring 1965
    Excerpt from Betty Lester, page 4
    FNS Quarterly Bulletin [3A]

Betty Lester writes:
    "The Trumpets Sounded"

"... At the bridge across the Middle Fork River, her horse, saddle empty and boots reversed in the stirrups, took up his position behind the hearse. Two couriers led him, and Anne Cundle in her riding uniform, walked beside him. Mrs. Breckinridge would have loved it." [3A]

— BETTY LESTER

I went to Wikipedia to explain the symbology of the boots.

"Traditionally, simple black riding boots are reversed in the stirrups to represent a fallen commander looking back on his troops for the last time." [10]

IN LIFE, Mary Breckinridge exhibited gracious hospitality, offering her Wendover properties for various holiday gatherings for the children of the community.

She hosted Christmas programs at the Garden House and Easter Egg hunts on the grounds of Wendover.

The Quarterly Bulletins have many entries about these special events. The Spring 1950 Quarterly Bulletin features a story about an Easter egg hunt on the riverbank of the Middle Fork River at Wendover. [3F]

The Autumn 1956, Autumn 1960, Autumn 1962, and Autumn 1979 Quarterly Bulletins are a few that include pictures of the Nativity Programs in the Garden House and of various individual participants. [3DA][3DB][3DC][3DD]

For more than half a century, the Nativity plays were held at Wendover, the staff having continued the tradition for decades after Mary Breckinridge's death. What wonderful memories were made by generations of Leslie County children. [3]

(A)(5)(C)(4)(3A)(10)(3)(3DA)(3DB)(3DC)(3DD)(3F)(B)(C)

22

SADDLEBAGS
CONTENTS

Did you ever wonder what was inside the saddlebags on the nurse-midwives' horses?

The following list is only a fraction of what the two compartments held:

- A pocket scale to attach to the baby's diaper to weigh him or her.
- Medication in bottles such as Castor Oil, Liquid Ergot, Mercurochrome, Morphine, Codeine . . .
- Silver Nitrate for the baby's eyes
- Cloth Diapers
- Supplies such as scissors, gauze, mercury thermometer, measuring tape, cord ties, shots, and various other items.[6]

23

FNS UNIFORMS

At FNS, it was fairly easy to tell the nurse-midwives and the Couriers apart.

While the Couriers typically wore white shirts and khaki pants, the nurse-midwives wore uniforms. [A]

In the summer, they wore those legendary blue uniforms of blue riding pants, riding boots, white shirts, ties, and blue vests. [2]

In the winter, they wore something a bit more appropriate for weathering the elements. Their winter uniform jackets were reminiscent of military attire. [2]

Both the summer and winter uniforms made the nurse-midwives easily identifiable to mountain people. [C]

Donna C. Parker writes:

"Nothing gave the appearance of a military organization more than the winter riding uniform. Reminiscent of Breckinridge's overseas garb, the FNS uniform was military in styling, differing primarily in the exchange of skirts for breeches . . . The hip-length coat fastened with a front-button closure and sported a medium-size collar and notched lapels. A self-fabric belt, characteristic of early twentieth-century clothing, buttoned over the coat. Large envelope pockets expanded when opened. A center back vent permitted the coat's skirt to spread as the nurse sat astride her horse. Nurses wore the tailor-made jacket and breeches with a white riding shirt, black four-in-hand tie, overseas cap, and knee-high boots. A comparison of the CARD uniforms . . . and the FNS uniforms . . . reveals the similarities in the jacket, shirt and tie, headgear, and footwear. The Frontier Nursing Service replaced the CARD insignia with the letters "F.N.S" embroidered in black on a self-fabric patch sewn to the upper portion of the left sleeve."
(11)

— DONNA C. PARKER

(A)(2)(C)(11)

24

THE OLD HYDEN HOSPITAL
GROUND-BREAKING, OCTOBER 1, 1927
DEDICATION: JUNE 26, 1928

- Built in 1927-1928 [3B, 3C]
- On October 1, 1927, construction on the old Hyden Hospital on Hospital Hill began when the cornerstones of the renowned building were placed by Mrs. S.C. Henning and Judge L.D. Lewis. [3B] [3S]
- Construction on the hospital was completed in 1928. [3C]
- On June 26, 1928, the dedication ceremony was held. [3C]
- For more on the laying of the cornerstone of the hospital, read the Quarterly Bulletin of the Kentucky Committee for Mothers and Babies, Inc, (Predecessor to the FNS.) November 1927 and Autumn 1970. [3B]
- For more on the dedication of the hospital, read the Quarterly Bulletin of the Frontier Nursing Service, September 1928. [3C]

The Maternity Ward:
(B)

- The maternity section of the old Hyden Hospital had two wards. The first ward consisted of four to five beds. The other ward was on the enclosed porch area and had two to three additional beds.
- In the early days of the old Hyden Hospital on Hospital Hill, expectant mothers were often times hospitalized for five to seven days after the baby came. While the mothers passed the time, waiting to go home, they sometimes completed tasks such as sewing boarders on receiving blankets and making baby gowns for the take home bundles.
- At the old Hyden Hospital, fathers suited up in hospital gowns before holding their babies, a practice that's still observed in today's modern hospitals.

OTHER TIDBITS:

- Following the practices set forth by Mary Breckinridge, new mother's were shown how to care for their babies before they were discharged.
- No matter if you had had ten babies already, you didn't leave the hospital until you were shown how to take care of the one you'd just had.
- You were shown how to bathe the baby, swaddle him or her, coached on feeding . . .
- The extended stay in the hospital after having the baby allowed the mother additional time to heal before being sent home.

DEDICATION: JUNE 26, 1928

(B)
   (3B)(3C)(3S)(B)

25

THEN VS NOW
FEES TO BIRTH BABIES

Let's look back in time to the late 1960s and early 1970s. In those days, the cost to birth a baby was an astounding fifty to one hundred dollars. And, in those days, those prices *were* astounding.

From oral history obtained from my mother, I know that in 1967, it cost $50 to have a baby at the old Hyden Hospital. That included prenatal and postnatal visits, as well as the actual delivery charge.

In 1971 and 1972, that fee was doubled at the same hospital, taking the total to $100 for the baby bill.

While those numbers may have been astronomical to parents in days of old, those babies they were taking home would go on to face fees in their own child-bearing years that no one could ever imagine. [B]

Today, in the United States, the average cost—without complications—to have a baby is just over $10,000. And, that's with insurance.

Factor in prenatal and postnatal care, and that cost rises to around $30,000. [1]

(B)(1)

26

FNS PROPERTIES
NATIONAL REGISTER OF HISTORIC PLACES

THERE ARE iconic Mary Breckinridge and Frontier Nursing Service properties in Leslie County. This is only a portion of them.

If you get a chance, be sure to visit them. Even if you can't go inside, make it a point to see where these local treasures are.

Wendover

- *The Big House on Wendover, which is now a Bed & Breakfast.* [1]
- *The Garden House*

ON HOSPITAL HILL

- *St. Christopher's Chapel*
- *The old Hyden Hospital*
- *Haggin Nurses Dorm*

AMY PENNINGTON BRUDNICKI

- *The Joy House*
- *Aunt Hattie's Barn*
- *Mardi Cottage*

Endnote 1

---

1. *At the time of publication, the Wendover Bed & Breakfast may have just closed permanently. That remains to be seen.*

27

THE MARY BRECKINRIDGE FESTIVAL

Every year that doesn't fall during a pandemic, on the first Saturday in October, the community comes together to celebrate The Mary Breckinridge Festival.

We celebrate our heritage and pay tribute to Mary Breckinridge by keeping her memory alive.

A riderless horse is the Grand Marshal of the parade, a nod to Mary Breckinridge and her lasting legacy.

The festival is steeped in rich mountain tradition. Booths are set up across town and range from food vendors, craftsmen, quilters, woodworkers, writers, seamstresses, jewelry makers, artists, informational booths, organizations, activities for the children . . .

The people of the Appalachian Mountains of Leslie County are a talented bunch, most of whom wouldn't be here, if not for Mary Breckinridge.

. . .

Every fall, a new Mary Breckinridge Queen is crowned, along with a Princess and little Princesses.

When you gather along the streets of Hyden to watch the motorcade of cars during the parade, you'll see many of them as they pass by.

A carnival always comes to town during the week leading up to the festival. It lingers into the night, as does live music, both of which are always great fun and reminiscent of another era.

28

NAMING OF WENDOVER

IN THE SUMMER OF 1926, it's said that Mary Breckinridge's Aunt Jane first coined the term, *Wendover,* when she was given the honor of naming the winding terrain. (7)

(7)

29

THE BIG HOUSE

NATIONAL HISTORIC LANDMARK

WENDOVER

RICH HISTORY of The Big House

In 1925, The Big House—a two-story log cabin, located on Wendover, Kentucky—was built for nurse-midwife, Mary Breckinridge. Once completed, invitations were sent out to every person in the county, requesting they attend an open house. Nearly five hundred people showed up, the majority of whom arrived on horseback. [A]

At the time, there were only five bathtubs in all of Leslie County, and two of them were in The Big House. [A]

With a bathtub on each floor, Mrs. Breckinridge offered the downstairs tub for the community to use. [8]

POST OFFICE

On November 15, 1926, the office area of The Big House was converted over and established as the first Wendover post office. The first Postmaster there was Martha Prewitt Breckinridge. [12] Also referred to as *Martha R.L. Pruitt* in another publication. [7]

If you visit The Big House today, you'll still see the interior mail-slot door that leads into the hallway where the post office was.

MARY BRECKINRIDGE

Up until her death in 1965, Mary Breckinridge drank her afternoon tea every day at 4pm. [A][3G] In earlier years, the tea was served in the living room area of The Big House. [A] Nearing her death in 1965, her tea was served in her bedroom. [3E]

She wrote her autobiography, Wide Neighborhoods, in The Big House.

Not only was Mary Breckinridge a writer and a published author, but she was also a great lover of literature. Visit her former home on Wendover, and you'll see shelf after shelf of well-worn titles filling the bookcases—collections that once belonged to her. [1]

HISTORIC LANDMARK

In 1991, The Big House was recognized as a National Historic Landmark. [A]

In 2001, The Big House was established as a Bed and Breakfast. You can go for a night's stay, an extended stay, or even just a hearty meal. [+]

The rustic charm of the nearly hundred-year-old cabin settles the soul and makes us proud to have such a local treasure right in our own backyards—one that we hope will be around for future generations to love.

For more interesting tidbits about The Big House, see the Autumn 1961 FNS Quarterly Bulletin. [3G]

ENDNOTE 1 (A)(8)(12)(7)(3G)(3E)

WENDOVER

1. At the time of publication, the fate of The Wendover Bed & Breakfast is unknown.

30

"DEDICATION OF LIGHTS"

DECEMBER 10, 1948

THE BIG HOUSE

The Big House

From 1925 to 1948, the only light source at Wendover was candles and oil lamps. When utility lines were finally ran in the late forties, Mrs. Roger Kemper Rogan, widow of former trustee and vice-chairman of the FNS, Roger Kemper Rogan, saw to it that resources were made available to the Frontier Nursing Service, providing electricity to all structures in her husband's memory.

Once the power lines were ran and connected, Mrs. Rogan, her sister, and Reverend Francis John Moore visited Wendover for the dedication.

On December 10, 1948, a dedication of light ceremony was held in the living room of The Big House.

THE BIG HOUSE

"The Living Room was filled with members of staff of the Frontier Nursing Service from its Hyden Hospital and its outpost centers as well as Wendover; and with a little group of mountain friends. At twilight, or as the mountaineers call it, 'the edge of dark,' Dr. Moore, in his robes, began to read the service which follows. (3U)(3V)

The shadowy living room was lit by candles and an oil lamp. When in his reading, Dr. Moore came to the words

'In Joyful Thanksgiving, we dedicate, at the edge of dark, these lights, to the Glory of God, to the dear memory of Roger Kemper Rogan, and to the service of this nursing community...'

When he came to these words, those who stood near the candles and the oil lamps extinguished them—those who stood by the first two electric lamps ever to shine in this remote forest turned on their greater light..."

(3U)(3V)

31

THE GARDEN HOUSE
NATIONAL HISTORIC LANDMARK
WENDOVER

- The original Garden House was built in 1931.
- In 1942, it was destroyed by fire. That same year, donations were raised, and another structure was built in its place—also called *The Garden House*. [A][3H]

THE GARDEN HOUSE has served many roles over the years:

- Dormitory for the Couriers
- Served as the Wendover Outpost Nursing Clinic and Administrative Building for the Frontier Nursing Service
- The basement of the Garden House served as host to the Christmas plays—also known as Nativity Pageants—for many decades.
- Various Wendover properties provide lodging to guests at the Bed & Breakfast—The Big House, The Barn, and The Garden House. [1]

FOR MORE ON the Garden House fire, read FNS Quarterly Bulletin, Winter 1942 [3H]

ENDNOTE 1 (A)(3H)

---

1. As stated previously, the fate of The Big House is unknown as the Bed & Breakfast has closed.

32

THE GARDEN HOUSE
CHRISTMAS NATIVITY PROGRAMS
WENDOVER

EVERY YEAR IN DECEMBER, children from the community came together to perform Christmas plays in the basement of the Garden House. The programs were called Pageants, Nativity Pageants, Nativity Plays, Christmas Pageants, and Christmas Plays.

I find that different generations referred to them by different names. (3DB)(D)

IN THESE PROGRAMS, the birth of Christ was portrayed by Leslie County children. The script was modeled after the Biblical story with baby Jesus in the manger, Mary and Joseph by His side, along with Angels, Shepherds, and Wise Men.

Speaking from experience, I will say this was a magical evening for many reasons. We performed the Christmas play, which was always great fun to dress up in the costume of the character we were portraying.

Once the play was finished, we had hot chocolate and cookies, prepared by Wendover staff.

The hot chocolate was creamy, chocolaty goodness, served in

small, styrofoam cups, and it was hotter than blue blazes. But, nearly fifty years later, I still hold cocoa to those same standards and would love to have the recipe from all those years ago.

After our refreshments, Santa always made a surprise visit to Wendover. The jolly old fella in the red suit welcomed us all and didn't leave until every child had a toy. We also received a paper sack filled with candy, nuts, and fruit.

As a child, I didn't put any thought into how this evening was funded. As an adult, though, I realize that this must have been quite an expense. From reading the Quarterly Bulletins, I understand that this program was carried out throughout the county, not just on Wendover.

Many of the bulletins state that thousands of children received toys at Christmas from FNS. It's my understanding that these toys were provided through donations to the Frontier Nursing Service.

Mary Breckinridge started this tradition shortly after the Frontier Nursing Service was founded. And decades after her death, the staff continued to carry on this tradition. In all, it ran for over half a century.

Just imagine all the children and parents who hold these special Christmas memories.

We may have grown up in one of the poorest regions in the commonwealth of Kentucky, but our heritage leaves us with memories that makes us rich beyond measure. This is why sharing our memories and experiences with the next generation is so important.

(3D_B)(D)

ST. CHRISTOPHER'S CHAPEL
CHAPEL WINDOW

HOSPITAL HILL

PHOTO BY ELBERT ESTEP

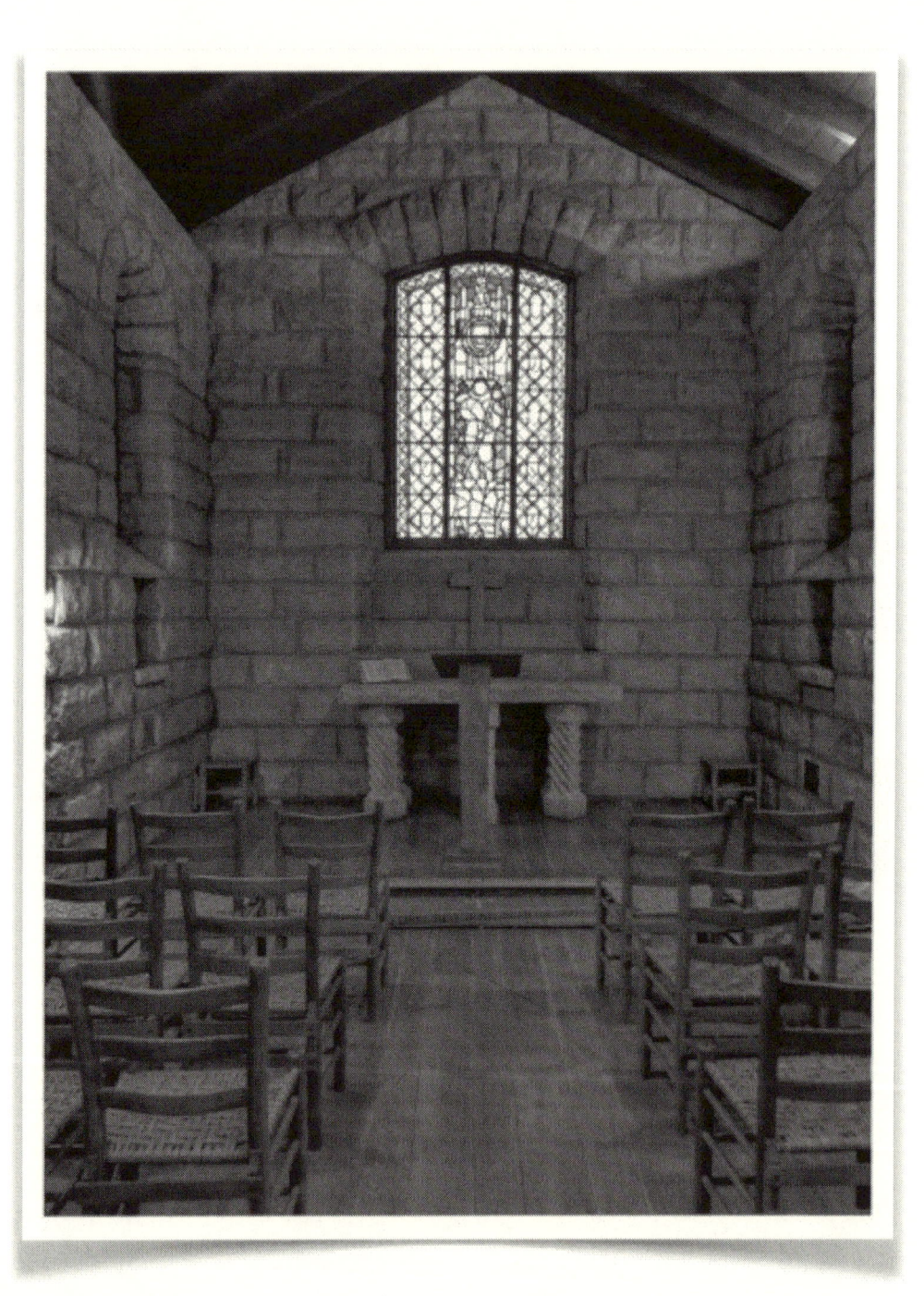

33

ST. CHRISTOPHER'S CHAPEL
NATIONAL HISTORIC LANDMARK

HOSPITAL HILL

THE WEE STONE HOUSE

IN EARLY 1960, the *Wee Stone House* was torn down on Hospital Hill to make room for a new building to be built on hospital grounds, the St. Christopher's Chapel. (3K)(3L)

ROGERS BEASLEY WRITES:

> "There had been considerable trepidation for some when first a bulldozer came on the site of the razed Wee Stone House three weeks ago. That Wee Stone House which sheltered the light plant for the Hyden Hospital has done its job long ago, and the site was to be cleared for another building to foster a more enduring light for the Frontier Nursing Staff and patients." (3L)

— ROGERS BEASLEY

CHAPEL CONSTRUCTION BEGINS

In April 1960, construction began on St. Christopher's Chapel on Hospital Hill in Leslie County. [3L] The little stone church was constructed from Appalachian timber and native sandstone by local craftsmen. [3]

The chapel was funded by donations. Not only did adults give money, but school-age children also pitched in. [3M][3N]

Inside the chapel, a wooden cross graces the altar. The cross was derived from a dogwood tree that was taken from the grounds of Wendover. [3O]

STAINED GLASS WINDOW

The chapel was built to house a beautiful 15th century stained glass window—a window Mary Breckinridge received as a gift from her cousin. [A]

The stained glass window depicts St. Christopher, the patron Saint of travelers, carrying the Christ child. [16]

ON AUGUST 19, 2020, the stained glass window was removed by Frontier Nursing University—the successor of the Frontier Nursing Service—and taken out of Leslie County.

THE PHOTO that leads up to this chapter is by my friend, Elbert Estep. In this photo, he perfectly captures the beauty of the chapel and the window that once graced the tiny structure.

FOR A MORE IN-DEPTH look at documentation on St. Christopher's Chapel, read the 1960 FNS Quarterly Bulletins—all four of them—and Winter 1961.

ST. CHRISTOPHER'S CHAPEL

. . .

(A)(3)(3K)(3L)(3M)(3N)(3O)(16)

34

THE UPPER SHELF
WENDOVER

IN DAYS GONE BY, there were several structures on Wendover that served as additional housing for FNS staff, guests, and residents. They were:

- The Upper Shelf
- The Lower Shelf
- The Wendover Cabin.

These structures no longer stand but have a rich history. [A]

ONE SUCH PROPERTY was the Upper Shelf. [1]

IT WAS SAID that there were one hundred and one steps that you had to climb to get to the single level, four-room cabin consisting of a living room, kitchen, dining room, and bedroom. [31)(A]

A fireplace in every room, each was equipped with a hob—a slotted iron bar frame with wide edges that was used to accommodate various items such as frying pans, tea kettles, popcorn poppers, or, when scooted to the edges, could be used as warming ledges. [31)(A)]

For more on the Upper Shelf, check out the Autumn 1944 FNS Quarterly Bulletin.
Endnote 1 (31)(A)

---

1. The Upper Shelf was torn down in 2010. It was located just before the Big House on the hill to the right.

35

MARY BRECKINRIDGE HOSPITAL

GROUND-BREAKING: OCTOBER 3, 1970

DEDICATION: JANUARY 5, 1975

GROUND-BREAKING CEREMONY

ON OCTOBER 3, 1970—on Mary Breckinridge Day—a ground-breaking ceremony took place with Mrs. Jefferson Patterson, National Chairman of the Frontier Nursing Service, laying the cornerstone for the new hospital, the Mary Breckinridge Hospital. (3S)

CONTENTS OF THE CORNERSTONE

In the Winter 1975 FNS Quarterly Bulletin, it is said that the cornerstone of the hospital includes some extraordinary items. They are listed as follows: (3W)

- "Mrs. Breckinridge's Bible
- A photograph of her son, Breckie, and her father, Major Clifton Rhodes Breckinridge
- The invitation to the dedication
- A list of all donors to the Mary Breckinridge Hospital

and Developmental Fund
- The object of Frontier Nursing Service from the Articles of Incorporation and the motto of the Service
- And a horseshoe in memory of bygone days
- Displayed on a silver tray presented the FNS by Mr. and Mrs. Roger L. Branham." (3W)

HOSPITAL DEDICATION

On January 5, 1975, a dedication ceremony was held for the new hospital, The Mary Breckinridge Hospital, named in honor for Mary Carson Breckinridge, a nurse-midwife who changed healthcare as we know it in Leslie County and in *Wide Neighborhoods* all across the nation. (3Q)

THE AUTUMN 1974 FNS Quarterly Bulletin gives an explanation as to why the hospital dedication was intentionally chosen to fall on January 5th—the eve of Old Christmas. (3R)

"January 6 is still remembered, in many areas of the Appalachian South, as Old Christmas, so it is perhaps appropriate that this important event in the history of the FNS and in the lives of Leslie Countians should come on the eve of a traditional holiday. Certainly the completion of and the move into the hospital is the nicest possible present for Christmas— old or new—that the FNS could possibly receive."

— FNS QUARTERLY BULLETIN AUTUMN 1974

(3S)(3W)(3Q)(3R)

36

OLD CHRISTMAS

OLD CHRISTMAS IS REFERENCED numerous times in the Quarterly Bulletins by Mary Breckinridge. As someone who seemed to place high importance on traditions, I think she would've been proud that the new hospital, named in her honor, was dedicated on the eve of such a special day.

ONE INSTANCE of Old Christmas being referenced in the quarterly bulletins was the Winter 1961 FNS Quarterly Bulletin.

> " . . . Even the children in the Kentucky mountains know about Old Christmas . . . It is only on the night of Old Christmas that the animals talk together in the barns and that the Christ child comes back to visit His world."

(3T)

37

FNS QUARTERLY BULLETINS
A TREASURE TROVE OF WONDER

THE QUARTERLY BULLETINS are filled with FNS news and happenings. [3]

DID you know you can do an Internet search for specific Quarterly Bulletins? Simply type in "FNS Quarterly Bulletin" and the timeframe you'd like to search. For example, "FNS Quarterly Bulletin, Autumn 1974."

Exploreuk.uky.edu is a good site for finding these. [9]

IN THE QUARTERLY BULLETIN'S, there's legal stuff and accounting info, if you're into that. But, if you take your time and scroll through each booklet, you'll find a treasure trove of wonder in each edition.

It's like opening a time capsule and a treasure chest, all rolled into one.

You just might read about your relatives or find a picture of yourself. Give it a gander. [3][9]

38

SPECIAL FNS HORSES

AT THE FRONTIER NURSING SERVICE, not only were the horses a functional and necessary means of transportation, but they were also well loved animals.

In the Winter 1958, FNS Quarterly Bulletin, Lucille Hodges notes some special FNS horses and interesting tidbits about each of them. Here's some excerpts of what she wrote:

"... Babette's going brings back memories of many other FNS horses.

• *Glen*, *from whose back I got my first glimpse of Wendover—around eight o'clock at night after almost a day with Mac at the Hyden Hospital. Marvin Breckinridge was there taking pictures and she was my guide.* (3JA)

• *Little Nell*, *the small mare used in teaching us beginners what was meant by the running walk.* (3JA)

• *Bruna that I was riding bareback when someone told me that the secretaries were not supposed to ride her.* (3JB)

• *Silver*, *rearing gently, her way of asking for a cone of ice cream at Hyden. (A treat for which "Harry" spoiled her)...*" (3JB)

REMEMBERING THE FRONTIER

— LUCILLE HODGES

For more on the FNS horses, read FNS Quarterly Bulletin, Winter 1958.

(3Ja)(3Jb)

39

"THE NIGHT BEFORE CHRISTMAS"

FNS QUARTERLY BULLETIN WINTER 1961, PAGE 12

BY BETTY PALETHORP, R.N., S.C.M.

"SHORTLY BEFORE 11:30PM on Christmas Eve, a little band of worshipers wended its way to St. Christopher's Chapel for a Carol Service. To those of us who had been fortunate to witness the birth and growth of the Chapel this was an especially happy occasion, for, to our Christmas joy was added glad participation in the first service to be held in St. Christopher's. It seemed particularly fitting that the beginning of this new life of prayer and praise should coincide with a celebration of the birth of our Lord and Savior.

The Chapel is beautiful, but the interior was even more lovely at Christmas due to the attractive figurines so kindly donated to St. Christopher's Chapel by an ex-staff member, Mrs. May Houtenville. They were placed underneath the stone altar and illuminated from behind.

About thirty-five people were present; a thrilling sight in church so late at night. We were very pleased to have a number of our Hyden friends, including Mr. Veley and Mr. Newell, our Presbyterian and Baptist ministers, in our midst to worship with us before the manger.

"THE NIGHT BEFORE CHRISTMAS"

The service was short, simple, and very reverent. After the opening carol, "Once in Royal David's City," Brownie said a prayer for the Chapel followed by a bidding prayer. Then came six carols, one of which, "Oh, Holy Night," was sung as a solo by Elaine Douglas, and interspersed were three readings of the Christmas Story given by Betty Lester, Molly Lee, and Anna May January. Then we recited the Lord's Prayer and the General Thanksgiving, and on the stroke of midnight the Chapel bell was joyfully pealed by Jinny Bramham aided by Molly Lee. With glad hearts we sang the thrilling Christmas morning hymn, "Christians, Awake, Salute the Happy Morn"; listened again to the Christmas Collect and heard Mr. Veley ask the Blessing. Finally we sang the most lovely Carol "Silent Night" and departed to our homes and beds. It was a happy Christmas for all. Our prayer is that the Chapel will be the source of many blessings both for those who use it for private meditation and for those who attend the daily evening service."

~FNS Quarterly Bulletin Winter 1961, page 12

40

"REFLECTIONS"

AUTUMN 1976 FNS QUARTERLY BULLETIN, PAGE 5 & 6

BY GOLDIE DAVIDSON

IN MY RESEARCH, I came across an article titled, Reflections, by Goldie Davidson. [3P] In the entry, you could feel the love she had for Mary Breckinridge and her mission, for the childhood memories Mrs. Davidson made on Wendover, and for the admiration she felt for the Frontier Nursing Service and the new hospital.

As I read her heartfelt words, I cried. I couldn't help it. Her gratitude for the work of Mary Breckinridge was simply heartwarming. I can't even begin to convey the emotion that she makes you feel.

It was such a well written and heartfelt entry, I've decided to include it in this book in its entirety. [3P]

GOLDIE DAVIDSON WRITES:

"Today I visited the new hospital here in Hyden. As I sit in the lobby, I noticed all the people passing back and forth—to see the doctor or to visit someone in the hospital, and I thought how good it was to know that we have such a nice place to go when we need some help. Someone from almost every family in the county would depend on the Mary Breckinridge hospital for some sort of care or help before a year is out.

Most people in this county knew Mrs. Breckinridge. She was the greatest thing that ever happened to us. Before she came and started the work at Wendover, people didn't have any way to get medical services. She loved all the people and wanted to help everyone. I can remember when families had no way of buying food and all they had to do was to go to Wendover and she would give them some kind of work which would help them feed their families. When a woman was expecting a baby, all she had to do was visit one of the FNS clinics and register and from then on she was closely attended as long as she needed care—and, in the beginning, the cost was only $5 or $10 for a new baby and a nice big layette.

Mrs. Breckinridge was concerned about all of her patients. I have seen tears in her big blue eyes when she was worried about a child sick—tears that she would wipe away on her apron. I can remember when she broke her back in a horseback accident but that didn't stop her for long. She was like a cowboy—after a time she was back on Teddy Bear, going about the job that needed to be done! One time when she came to our house to visit it was so cold that her feet were frozen to the stirrups and daddy had to take a hammer to break the ice before she could get off the horse. She went through [heck] and high water for people here in this county and left a trail behind her, showing the good she had done. There is Wendover, and the old Hyden Hospital, and all the outpost centers, still helping people every day—doing all they can for us. Now let us try to help the FNS.

I remember when a nurse would be called out for a home delivery. She would stay all night and into the next day to make sure the mother and baby were safe—and she would cook and help with the other children while she was waiting for the mother to deliver the new baby. Nurses have played a big part in our lives and I know many of us remember this. These are good memories.

At Christmastime Santa Claus would visit everyone in the community, sometimes at the pageant at Wendover, sometimes on a sled drawn by "Old Blue", the Wendover mule. At Easter, we would all go to Wendover for our annual egg hunt, with Mrs. Breckinridge there to see that we had a good time, and to touch us all before we left. FNS made it possible for the young girls in our community to learn to sew and knit and quilt and helped us make clothing for school—and there was hot chocolate and cookies at the end of the classes because Mrs. Breckinridge said this will keep us warm on the way home. I can remember going with her to feed her chickens when I would carry her basket and help gather eggs. Once, on a winter day, when my father had to go to the clinic at Wendover, Mrs. Breckinridge was afraid he was cold so she found him an overcoat and a wool scarf and buttoned him up herself so he would be warm on the way home.

You don't forget things like that easily. It wasn't just my family—most of the older people who were here could tell how the FNS has helped them and their families. Many of us will remember others at Wendover—Agnes Lewis, Lucile Hodges, Betty Lester who is still with us in Leslie County and loved by everyone. There were Jahugh Morgan and his wife, Belle, and Lee Morgan, and Hobert Cornett who all spent many years at Wendover. I wish I could remember them all because they were good, faithful workers.

I wondered what in the world we would have done without our hospital. Anyone who has not taken the time to visit the new hospital should do so and see what is being done there. One day I walked into one of the rooms and saw an old lady holding the hand of her son who was dying. If he had had to go to Harlan or Hazard or Lexington, she would not have been able to be with him and comfort him in the short time he had left. Sometimes we grumble and complain about things at the hospital but we always go back when we need help!

The FNS needs our help now to continue to serve us. If each of us gave a small amount in remembrance of all the joy that has come to us from FNS, it would be a large amount for FNS and would mean a better Christmas for us all." (3P)

— GOLDIE DAVIDSON

(3P)

41

HERITAGE

FIVE GENERATIONS of my family have known and loved The Big House and the legacy of Mary Breckinridge.

Mary Breckinridge, her nurse-midwives, and her couriers have deeply impacted my family.

Because of her mission, many members of my family are saddlebag babies, FNS babies, have become nurses, healthcare workers, and became committee members affiliated with Wendover and FNS.

FIVE GENERATIONS. That's some deep roots and deep connections.

THE OLDER GENERATIONS were friends with Mary Breckinridge, her Nurse-Midwives, and the Couriers. The younger generations formed lasting friendships with staff members at Hospital Hill and Wendover.

My family has spent time at Wendover—some even having tea with Mary Breckinridge. Others have worked there, ate meals in the Dog Trot Dining Room, the main dining room, the kitchen, made friends at Wendover, had overnight stays, and made lasting memories.

When Mary Breckinridge passed away in 1965, my family mourned her death and attended her funeral.

But, all of Leslie County did.

In days gone by, the nurse-midwives and couriers spent a great deal of time visiting my family members on Hurricane Creek and sharing meals with us.

They were like family.

My family has a story that's so similar to all of yours. We all love and cherish Wendover, Hospital Hill, FNS, Mary Breckinridge, and her mission.

To some, The Big House is just a building, and Wendover, just another country lane. But to my family, and to all of Leslie County, it represents so much more.

It's our heritage. It's our legacy. It's who we are.

42

PRESERVING HISTORY

THIS BEARS REPEATING: Leslie County is deep-rooted in the legacy of Mary Breckinridge and the Frontier Nursing Service. Let's make it *our* mission to pass along stories to future generations who will never experience her work firsthand, but who wouldn't be here if not for her.

WHO CAN you tell about the legacy of Mary Breckinridge?

IF YOU'D LIKE to know more about Mary Breckinridge, Leslie County has many wonderful historians.

I recommend contacting Michael Claussen. michaeljky@gmail.com His knowledge of Mary Breckinridge and the Frontier Nursing Service is unsurpassed. He's a tremendous asset to Frontier history.

Make it a point to get with a frontier historian, to learn from them, to listen to them, before it's too late . . .

THE BIG HOUSE

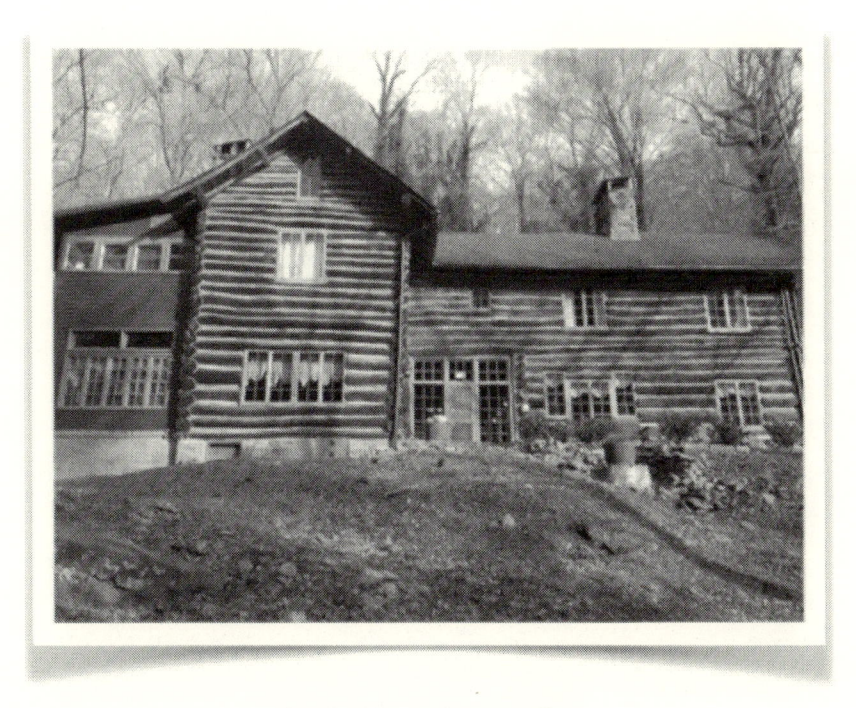

Photo by Kim Pennington Huffman

43

MARY BRECKINRIDGE'S CANES & WALKING STICKS

PHOTO BY AMY PENNINGTON BRUDNICKI

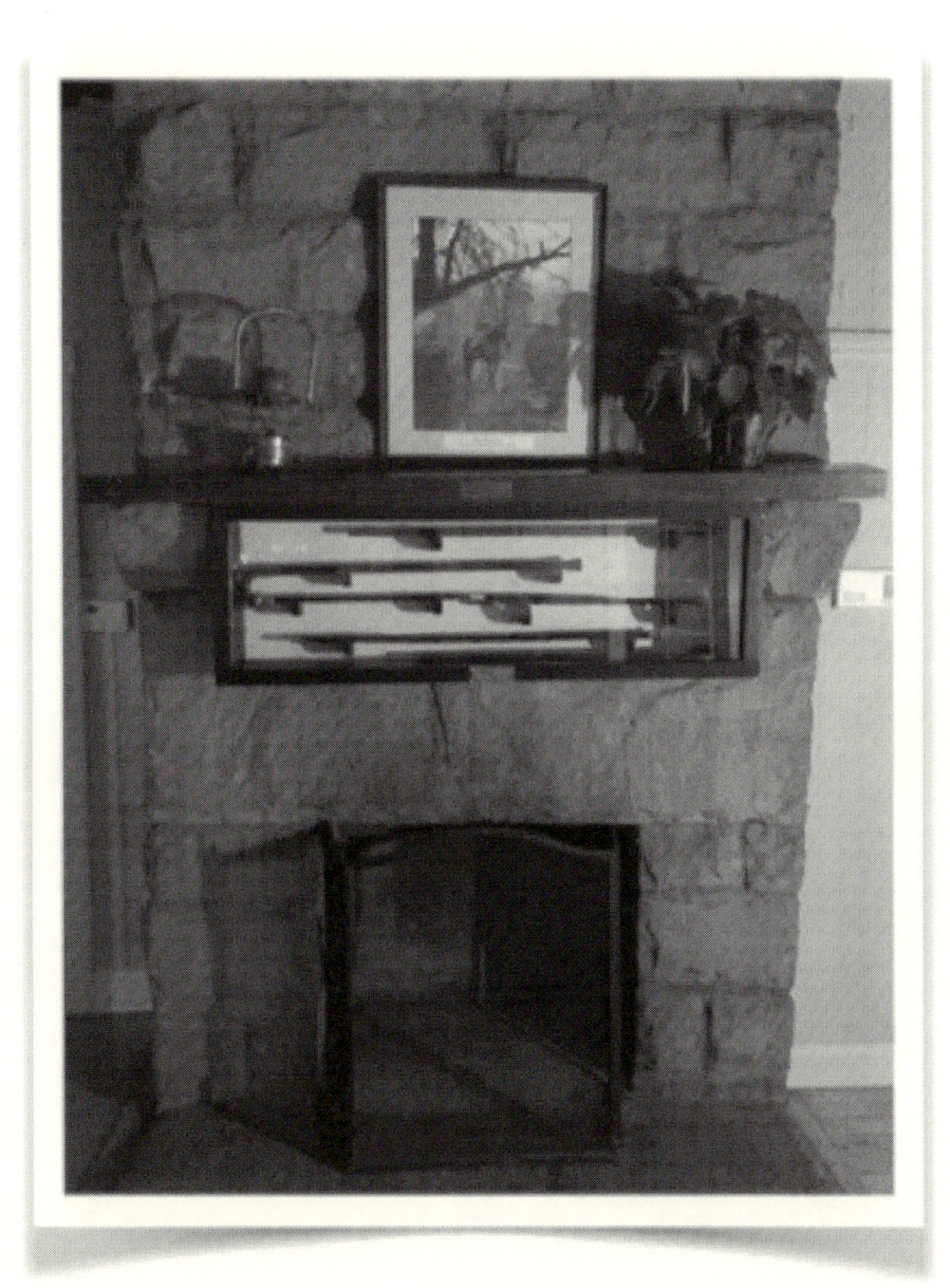

44

BEAUTIFUL CHINA
IN DOG TROT DINING ROOM

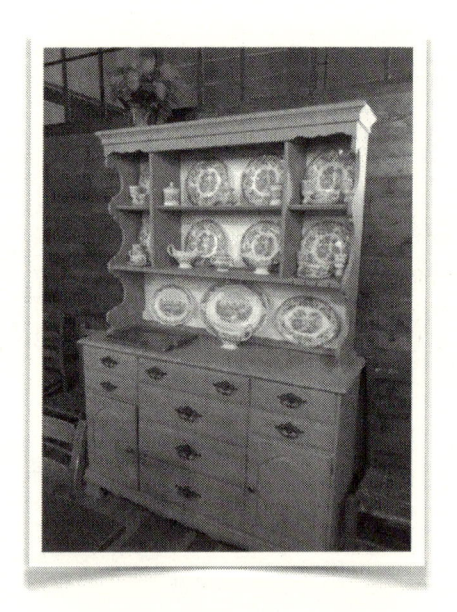

Photo by Kim Pennington Huffman

45

CHRISTMAS PLAY
AT THE WENDOVER GARDEN HOUSE

1975

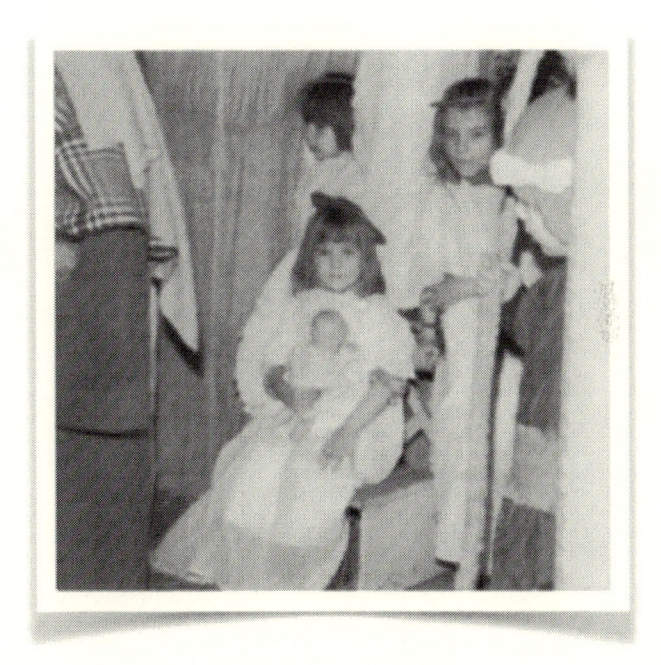

Amy Pennington Brudnicki

46

FIFTH GENERATION MAGGARD
ENJOYING WENDOVER

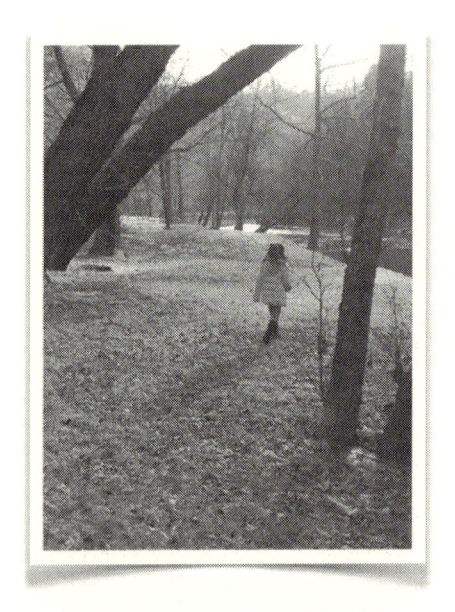

Photo by Amy Pennington Brudnicki

47

DAYS GONE BY
A BULGING SADDLEBAG

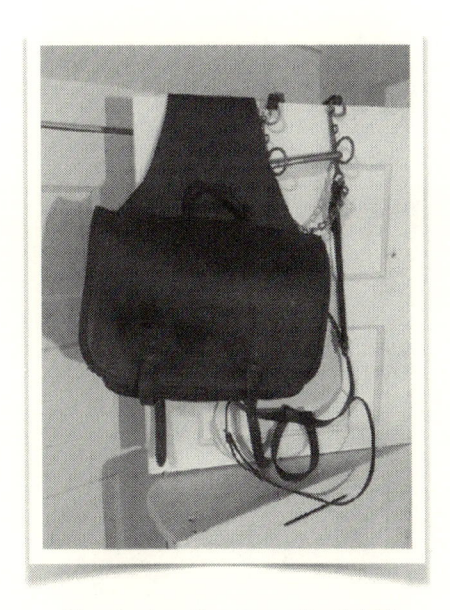

Photo by Amy Pennington Brudnicki

48

"A CURB BIT HANGS SILENTLY,

LONG SINCE HEARING THE SOUND OF BOOTSTEPS COMING TO SADDLE A MOUNT FOR A DAY'S RIDE."

QUOTE BY AUDREY MAGGARD CLOWERS

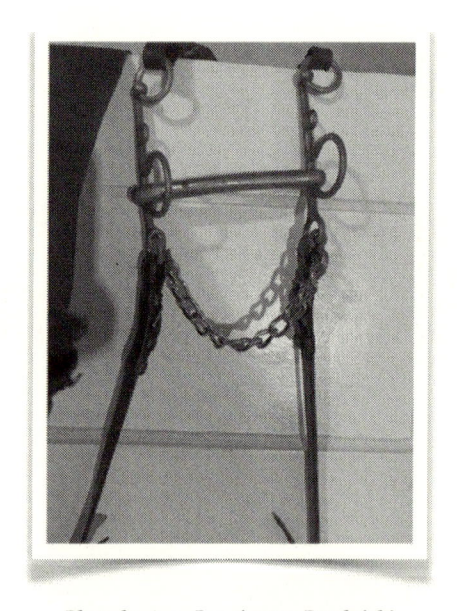

Photo by Amy Pennington Brudnicki

49

THE UPPER SHELF
LODGING FOR FNS STAFF

PHOTO TAKEN 2010

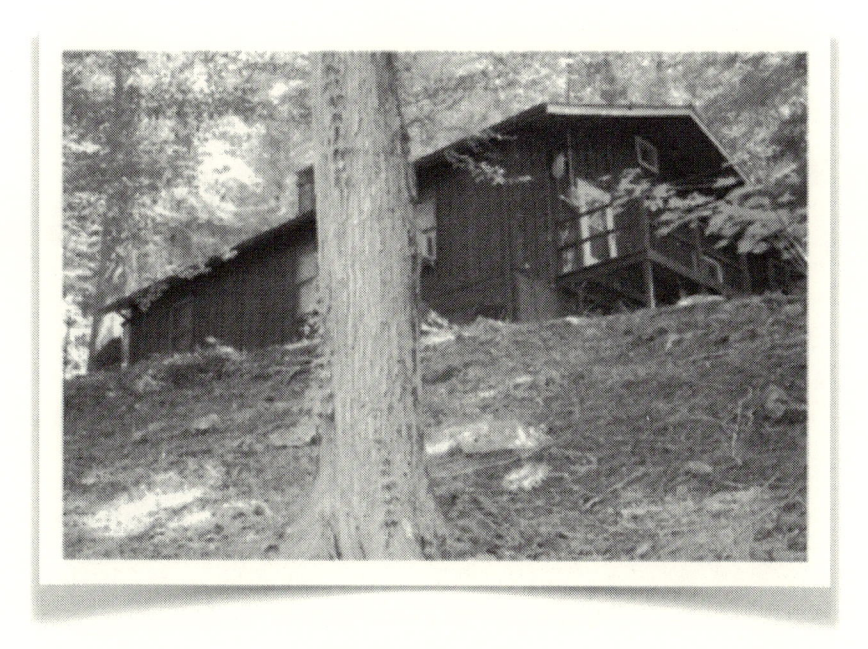

Photo by Michael Claussen

50

VINTAGE BOOKS & BOOKCASES
A SMALL SAMPLE OF MARY BRECKINRIDGE'S PERSONAL COLLECTION OF BELOVED BOOKS

THE BIG HOUSE LIVING ROOM

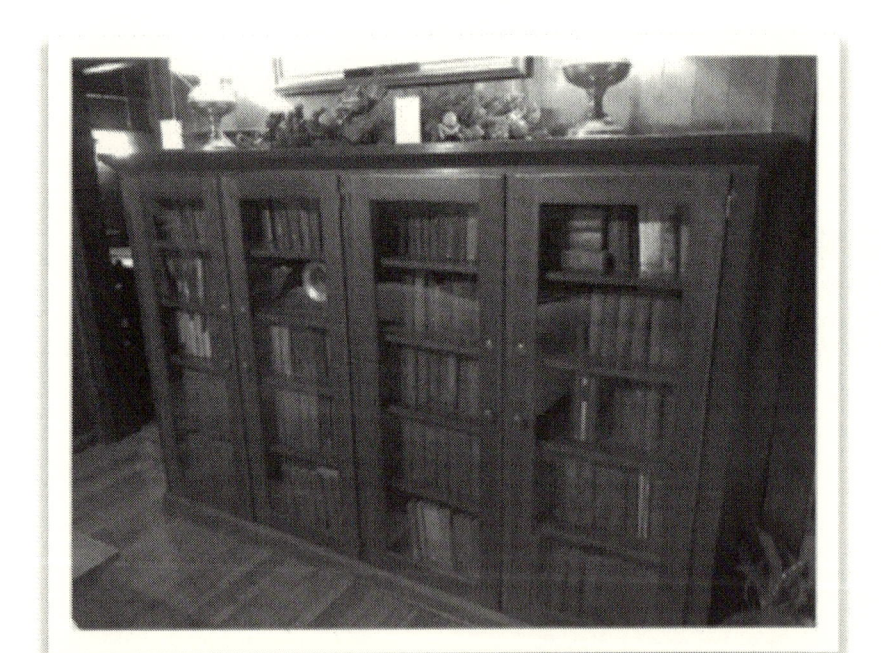

Photo by Kim Pennington Huffman

51

BOOK SIGNING
AT THE BIG HOUSE
SEPTEMBER 21, 2019

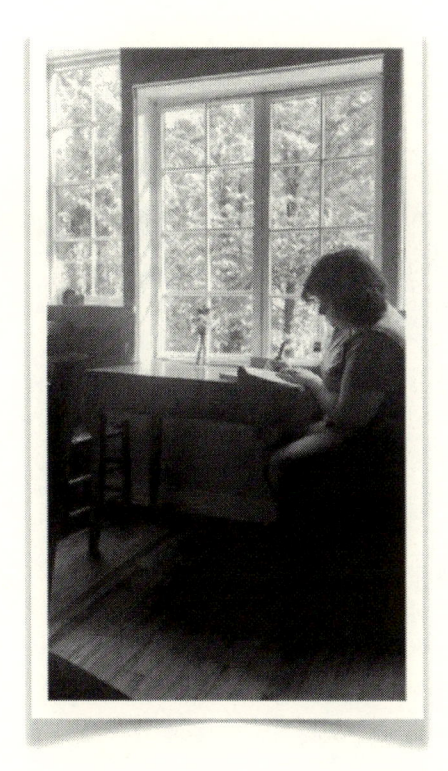

Photo taken of Amy Pennington Brudnicki by Wendy Collett

52

MARDI COTTAGE
HOSPITAL HILL

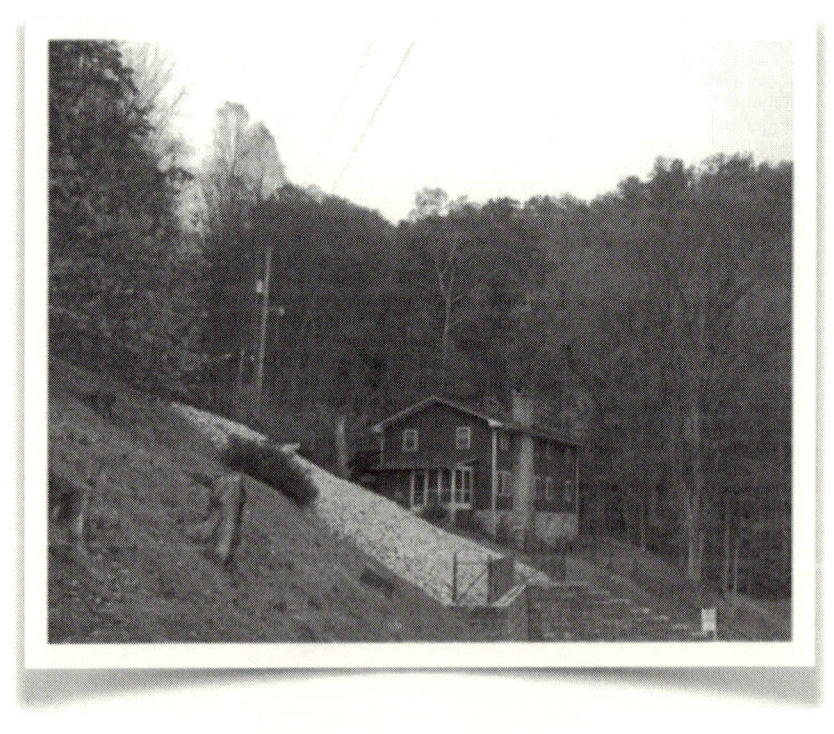

Photo by Amy Pennington Brudnicki

53

HAGGIN NURSES DORM
HOSPITAL HILL

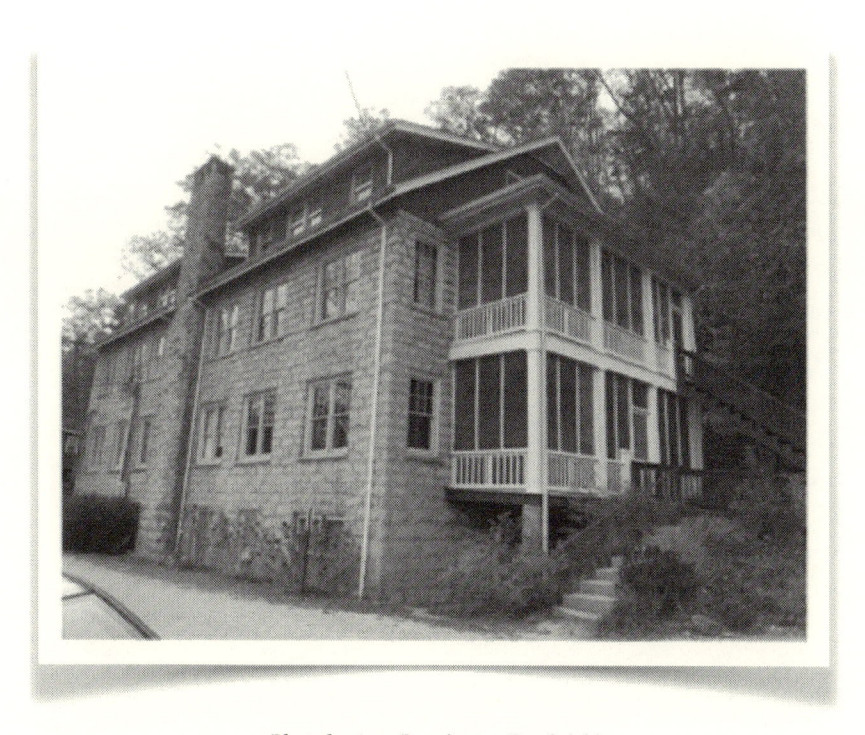

Photo by Amy Pennington Brudnicki

54

STONE STEPS
HOSPITAL HILL

PHOTO TAKEN 2018

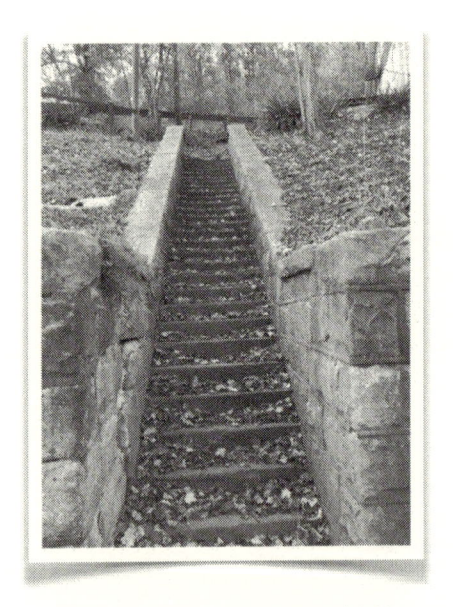

Photo by Amy Pennington Brudnicki

55

FOLLOWING IN THE STEPS OF MARY BRECKINRIDGE,
PEGGY LOVETT COVEY BECAME A REGISTERED NURSE

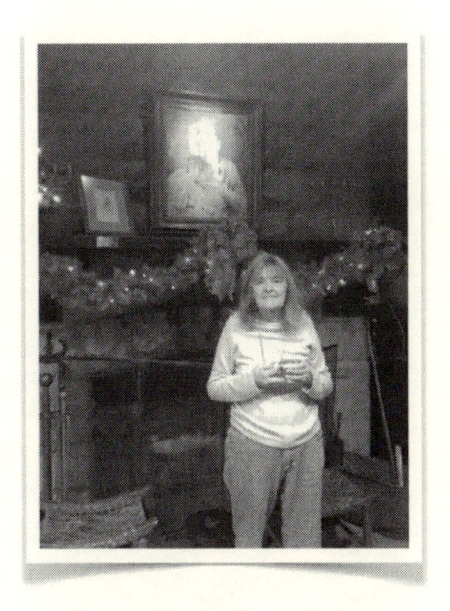

Photo by Kim Pennington Huffman

STONE STEPS
TO THE BIG HOUSE
OCTOBER 2015

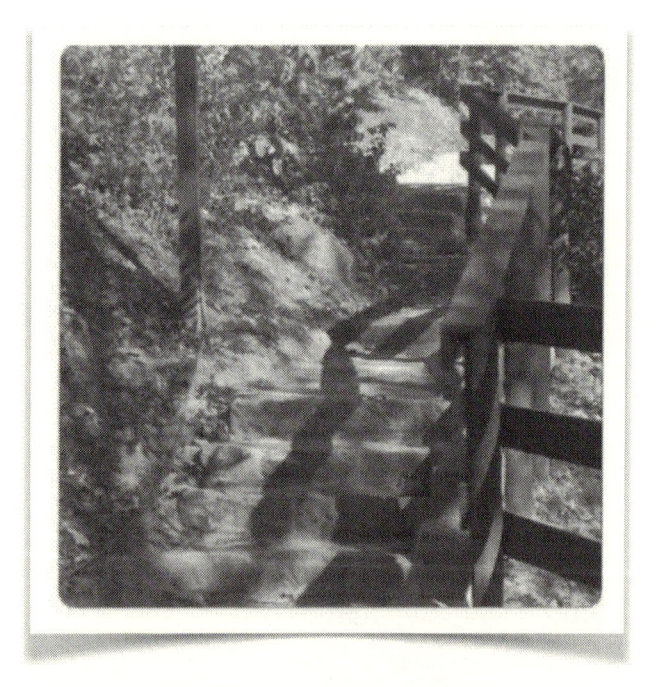

Photo by Amy Pennington Brudnicki

57

WENDOVER
BED & BREAKFAST SIGN

OCTOBER 17, 2020

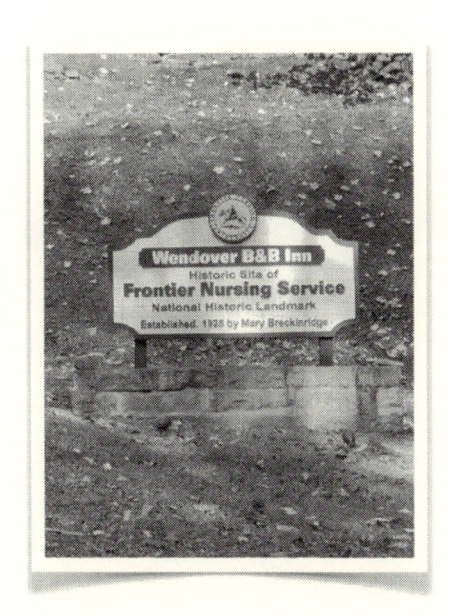

Photo by Amy Pennington Brudnicki

58

ROCK WALL
BEHIND THE BIG HOUSE

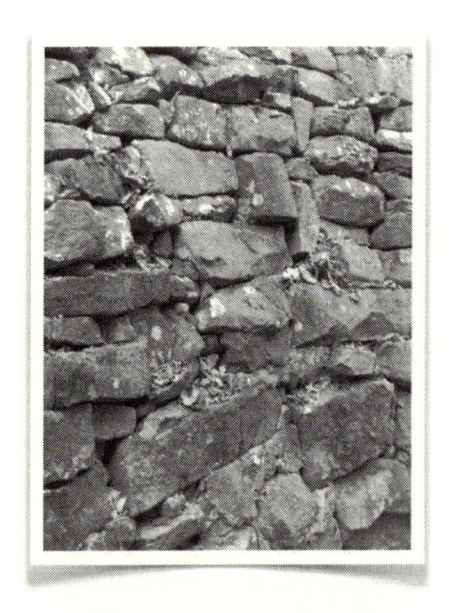

Photo by Amy Pennington Brudnicki

59

PICTURESQUE GROUNDS
AT WENDOVER

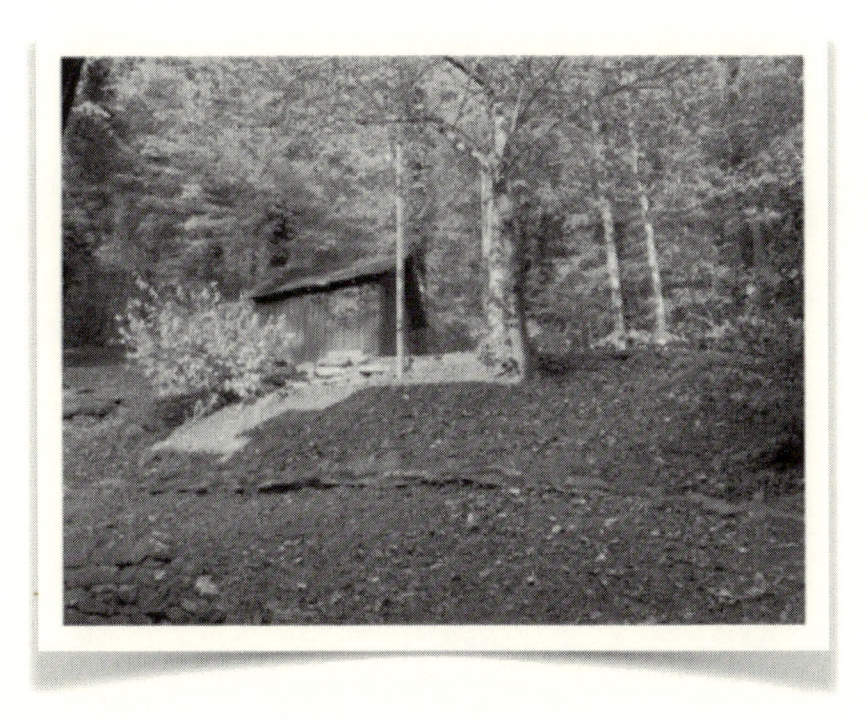

Photo by Amy Pennington Brudnicki

60

THE BIG HOUSE
FROM WENDOVER ROAD
DECEMBER 2017

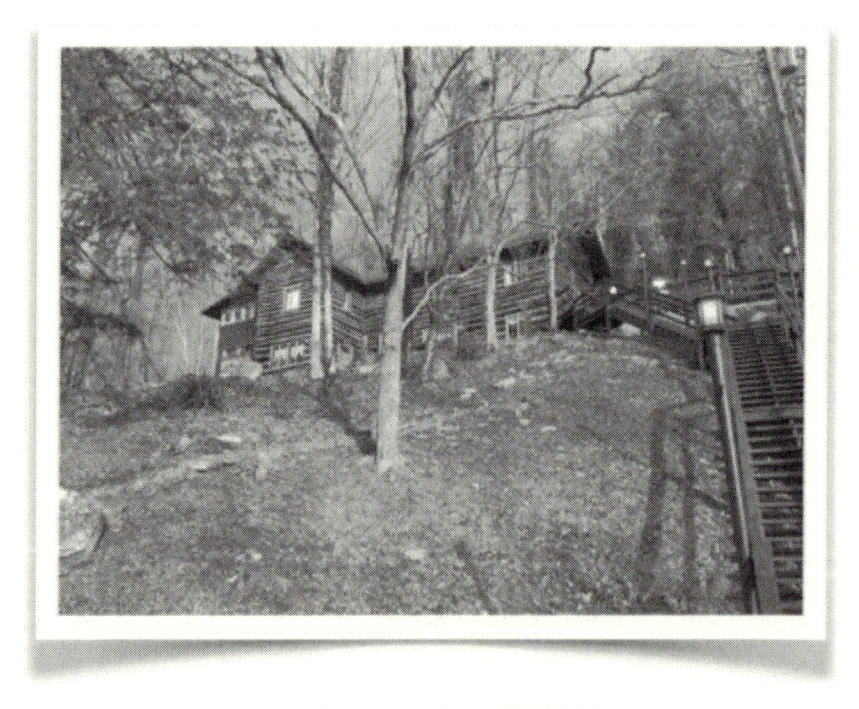

Photo by Amy Pennington Brudnicki

61

RIVERBANK
AT WENDOVER

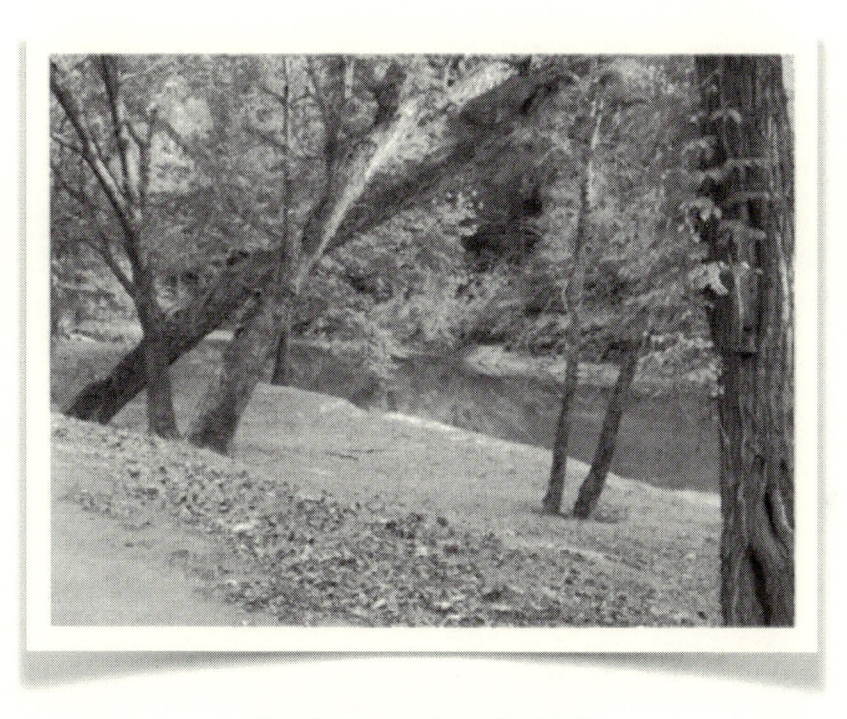

10/17/2020

Photo by Amy Pennington Brudnicki

62

ROCKY RIVERBED
AT WENDOVER

10/18/2015

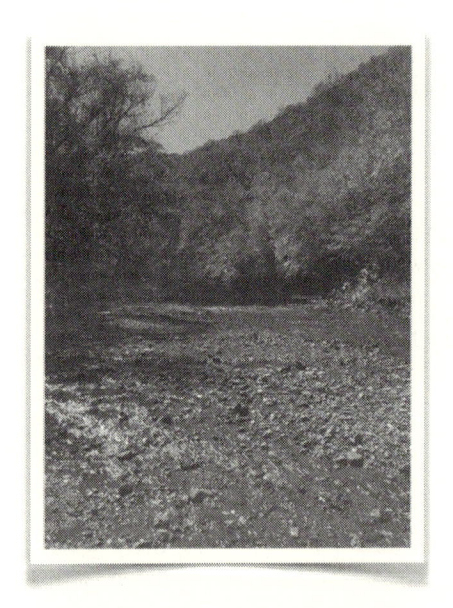

Photo by Amy Pennington Brudnicki

63

ST. CHRISTOPHER'S CHAPEL
ENTRYWAY

HOSPITAL HILL

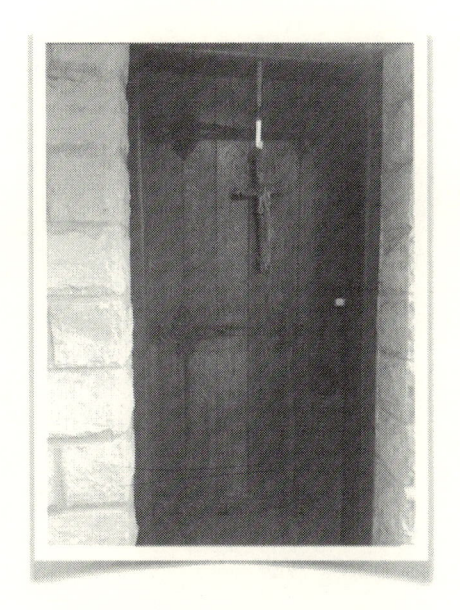

Photo by Amy Pennington Brudnicki

64

ST. CHRISTOPHER'S CHAPEL
HOSPITAL HILL

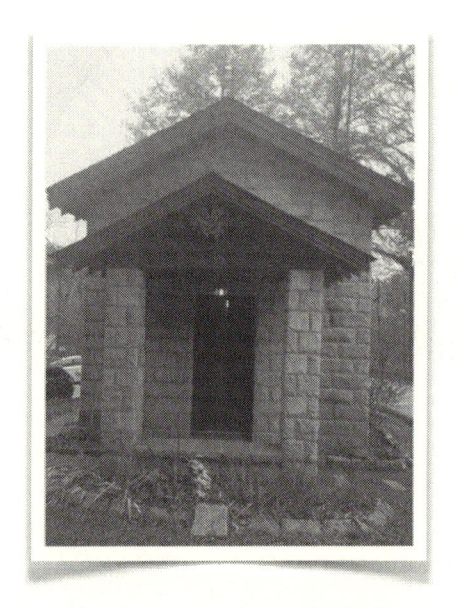

Photo by Amy Pennington Brudnicki

VINTAGE BOOKS
ST. CHRISTOPHER'S CHAPEL
HOSPITAL HILL

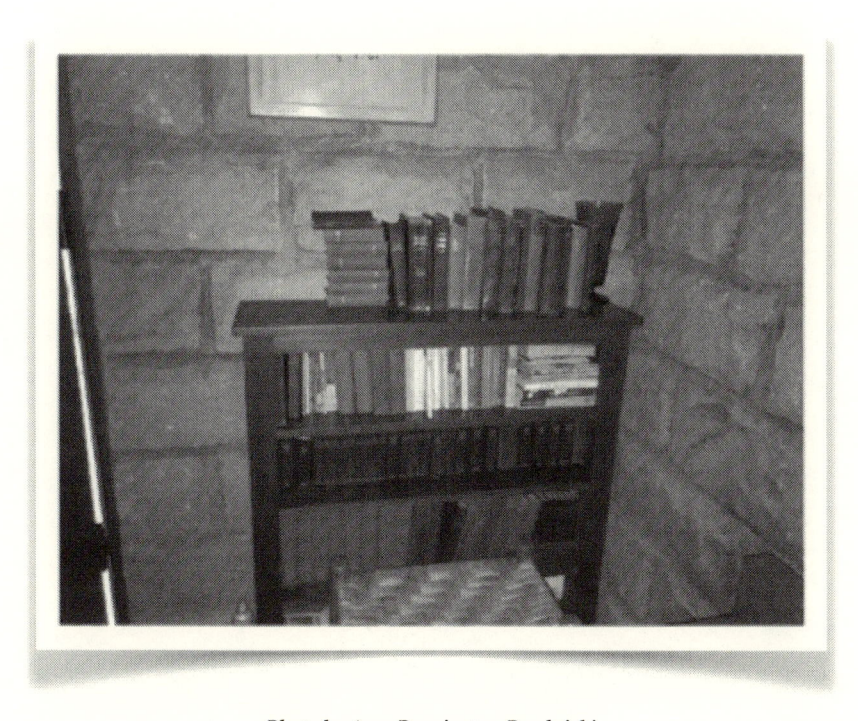

Photo by Amy Pennington Brudnicki

66

ORGAN
INSIDE ST. CHRISTOPHER'S CHAPEL
HOSPITAL HILL

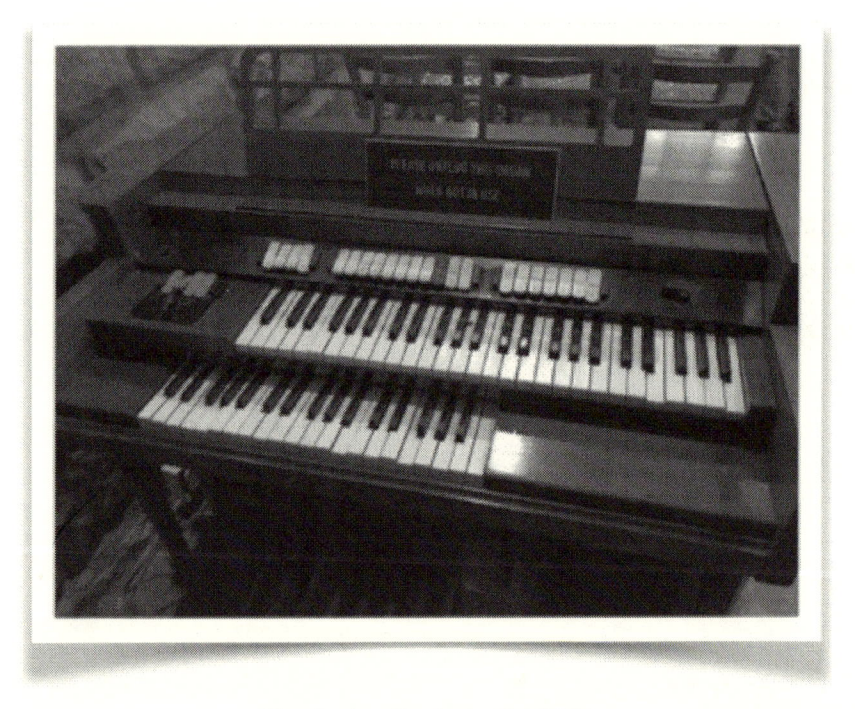

Photo by Amy Pennington Brudnicki

67

CHRISTMAS PLAY
AT WENDOVER GARDEN HOUSE

1975

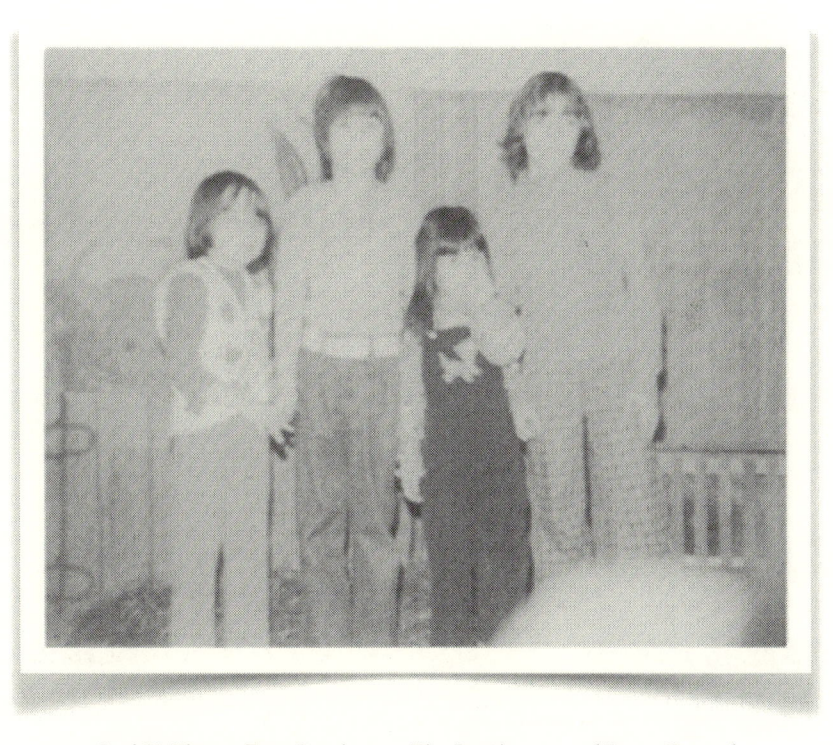

Lori McKinney, Tony Pennington, Kim Pennington, and Roger Howard

68

ENCLOSED PORCH
OFF LIVING ROOM OF THE BIG HOUSE

DECEMBER 14, 2018

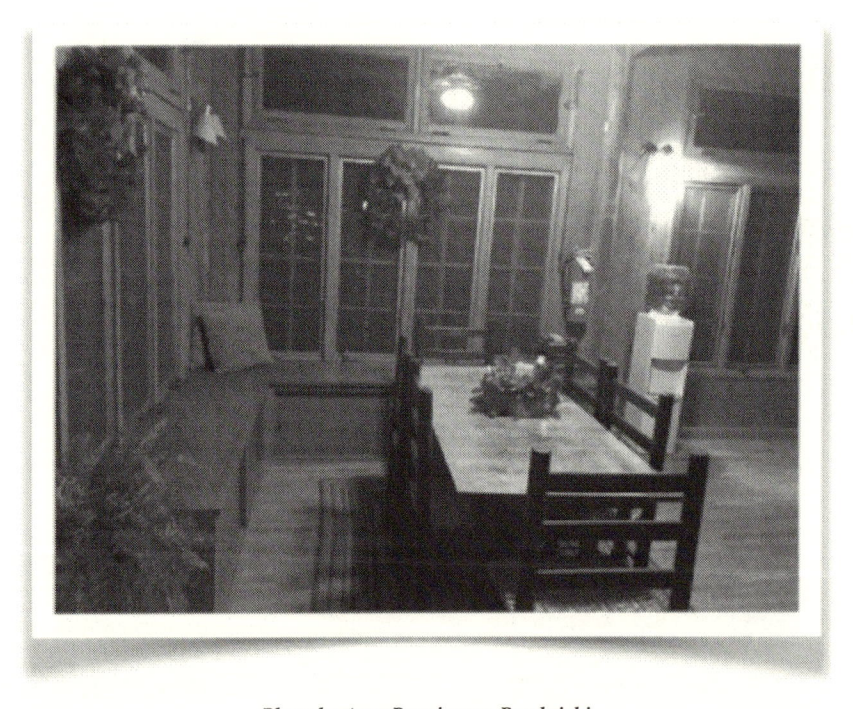

Photo by Amy Pennington Brudnicki

69

WENDOVER CHRISTMAS PLAY
THE GARDEN HOUSE

1975

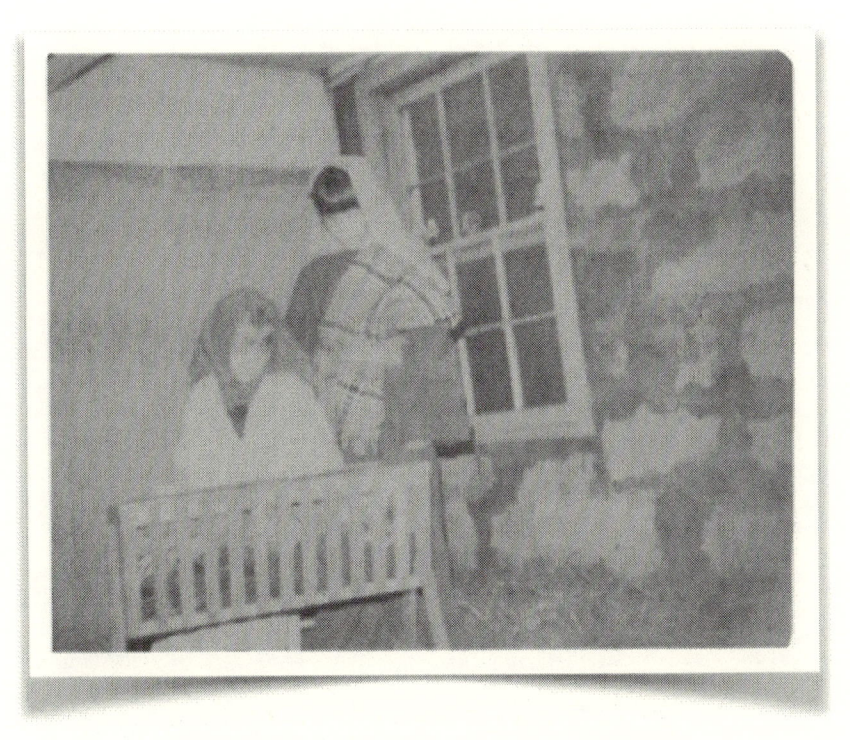

Tina McKinney & Tony Pennington as Mary & Joseph

70

THE DOG TROT DINING ROOM
LOGS SOURCED FROM LOCAL TIMBER

PHOTO TAKEN DECEMBER 14, 2018

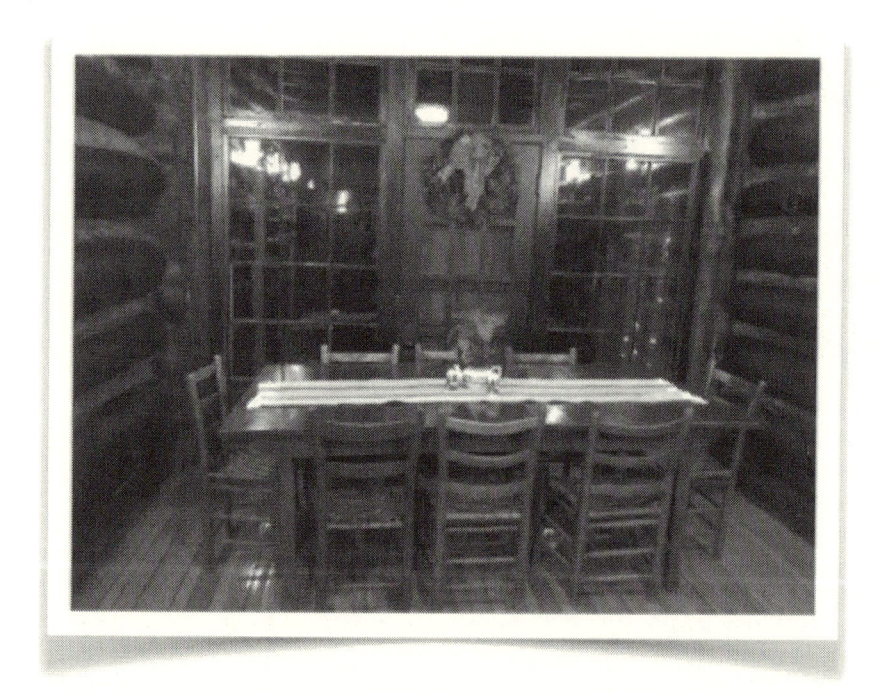

Photo by Amy Pennington Brudnicki

71

THE FRONT DINING ROOM
THE BIG HOUSE

12/14/2018

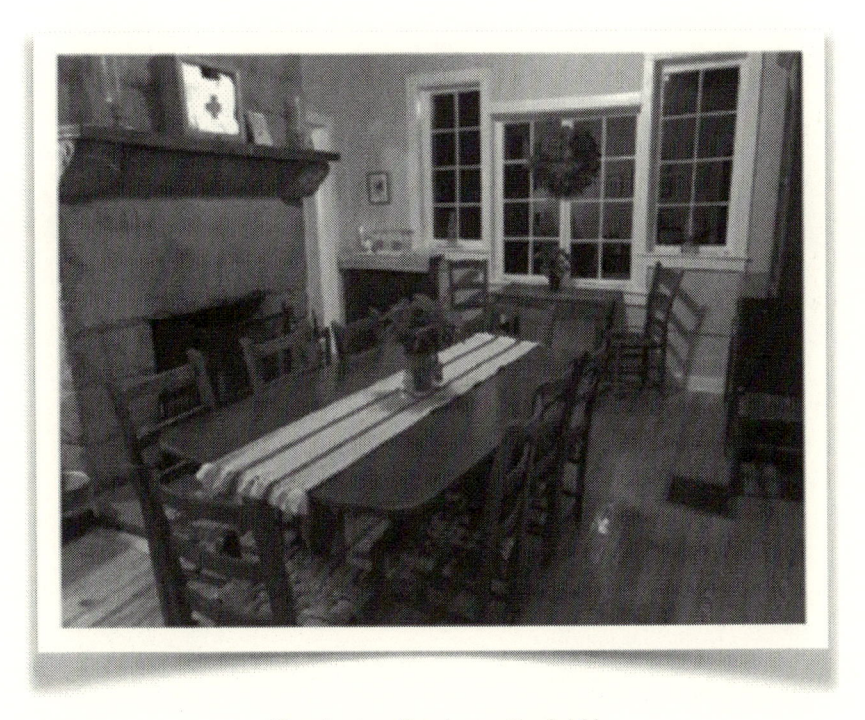

Photo by Amy Pennington Brudnicki

72

THE FRONT ROOM
THE BIG HOUSE

DECEMBER 14, 2018

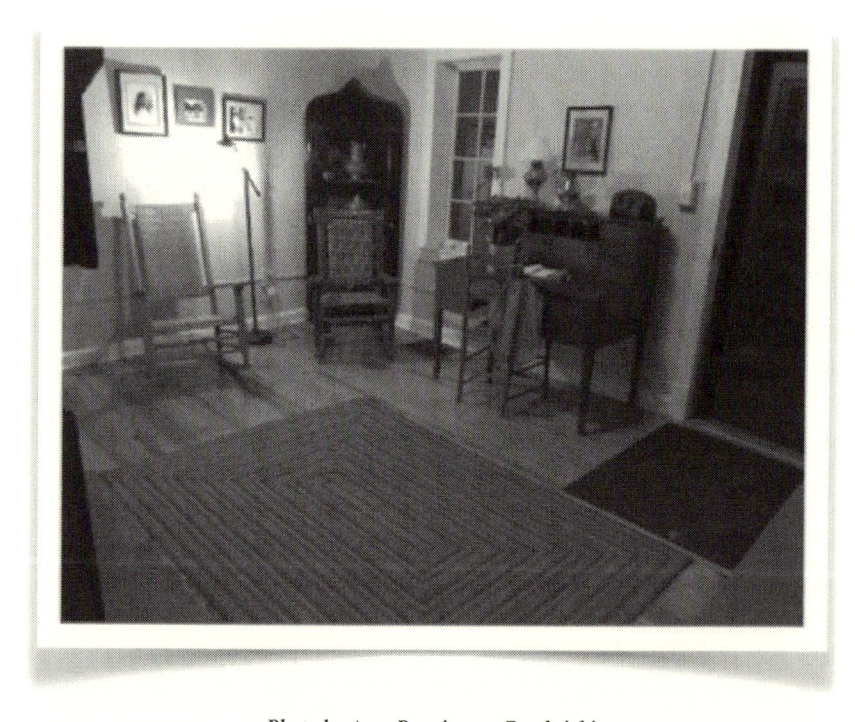

Photo by Amy Pennington Brudnicki

73

NATIVITY PLAY
AT THE GARDEN HOUSE

1975

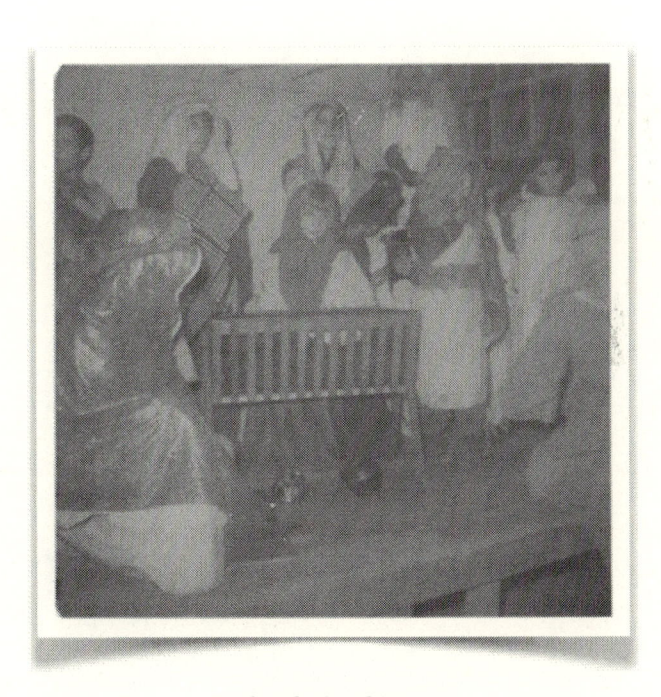

Photo by Hazel Lovett

74

CHRISTMAS TREE IN THE LIVING ROOM OF THE BIG HOUSE

DECEMBER 27, 2019

PHOTO BY AMY PENNINGTON BRUDNICKI

CHRISTMAS TREE IN THE LIVING ROOM OF THE BIG HOUSE

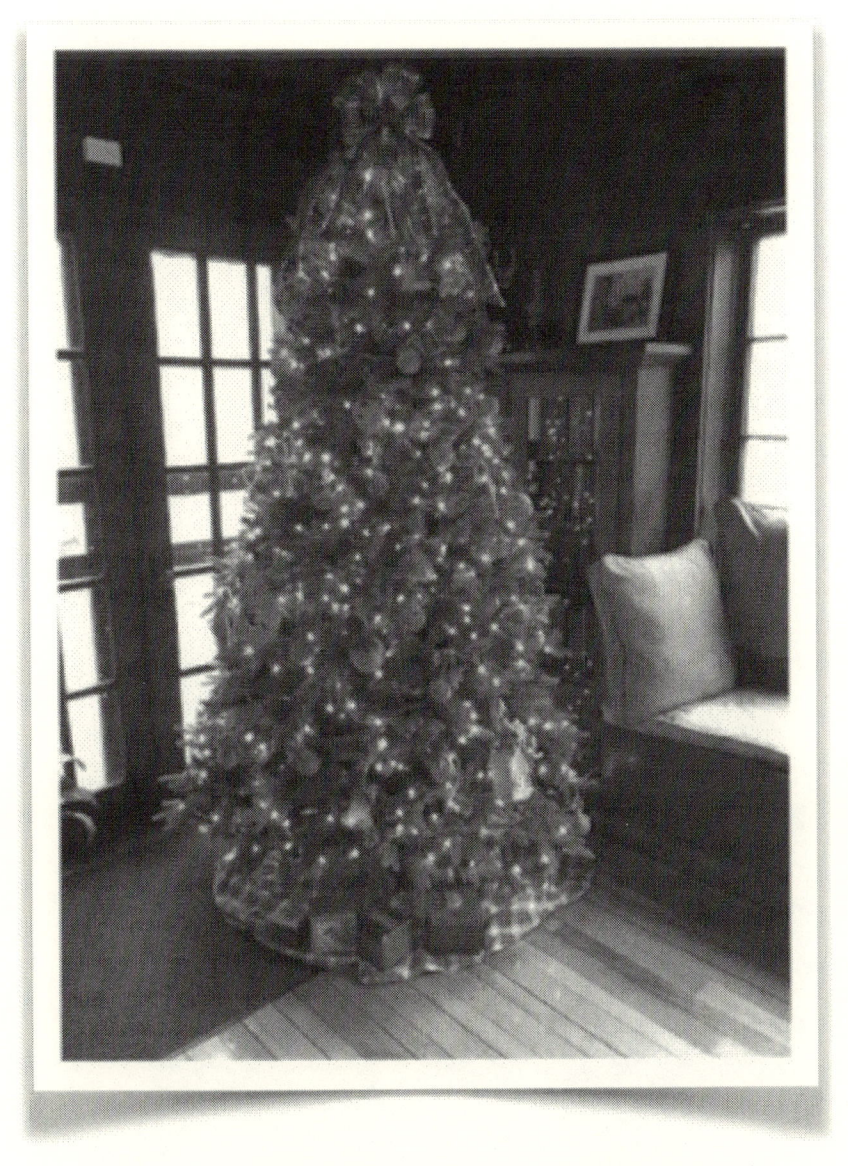

I've spent many holiday season's visiting Wendover. It holds a special magic of Christmas that I simply cannot explain.

75

BEAUTIFUL FIREPLACE
CRAFTED FROM LOCAL SANDSTONE

PHOTO TAKEN DECEMBER 2017

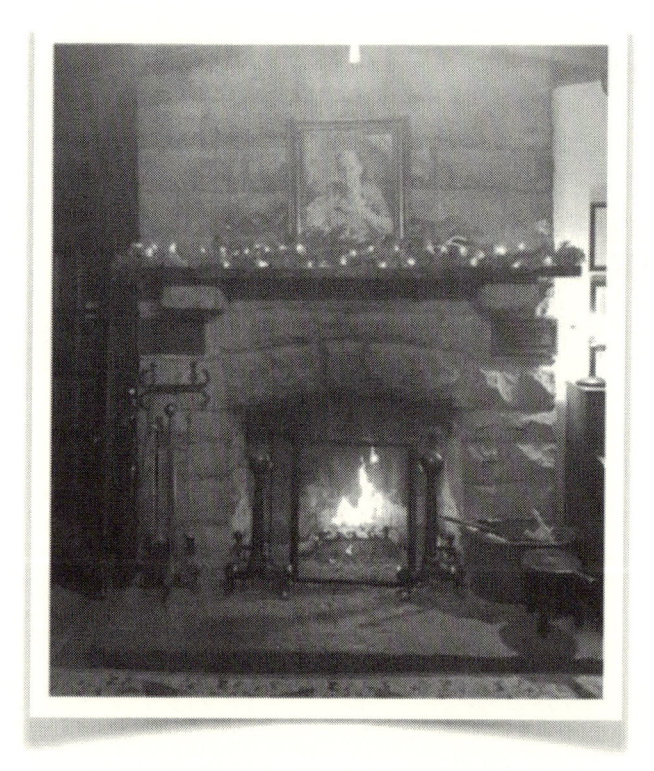

Photo by Amy Pennington Brudnicki

76

STAIRCASE
THE BIG HOUSE
DECEMBER 27, 2019

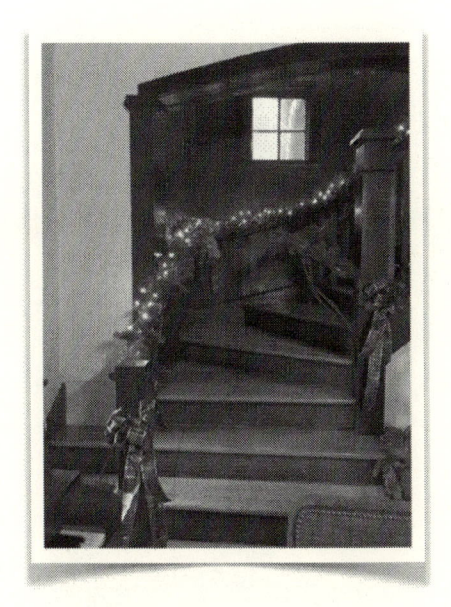

Photo by Amy Pennington Brudnicki

77

LIVING ROOM WINDOW
THE BIG HOUSE

HILLSIDE OVERLOOKING THE MIDDLE FORK RIVER

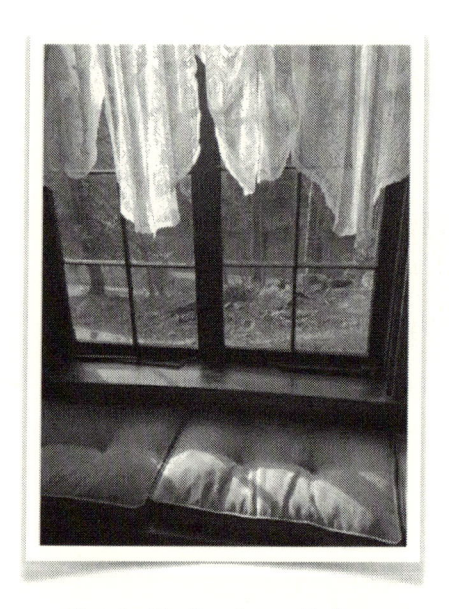

Photo by Kim Pennington Huffman

78

THE DOG TROT DINING ROOM
THE BIG HOUSE
OCTOBER 2015

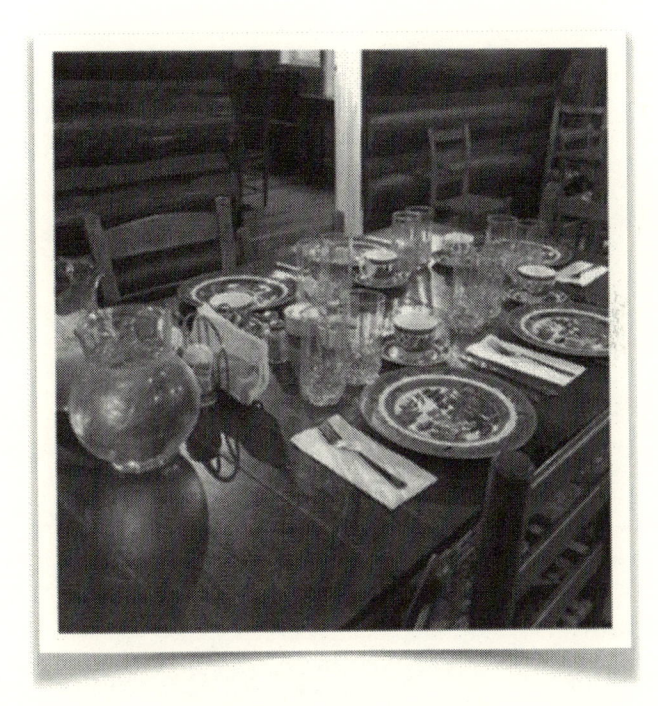

Photo by Amy Pennington Brudnicki

79

WENDOVER NATIVITY PLAY
THE GARDEN HOUSE

1975

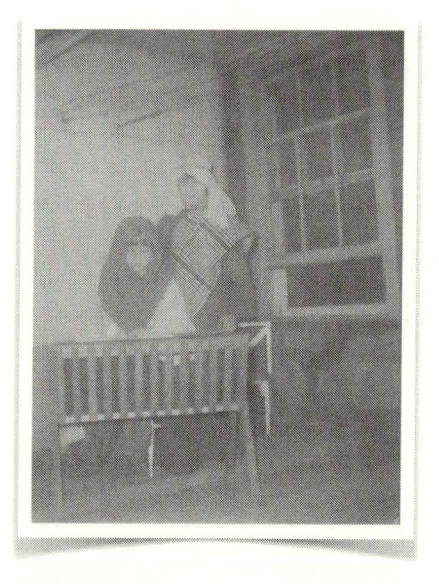

Tina McKinney and Tony Pennington as Mary & Joseph

80

THE MANGER
FROM THE CHRISTMAS PLAYS
OCTOBER 17, 2015

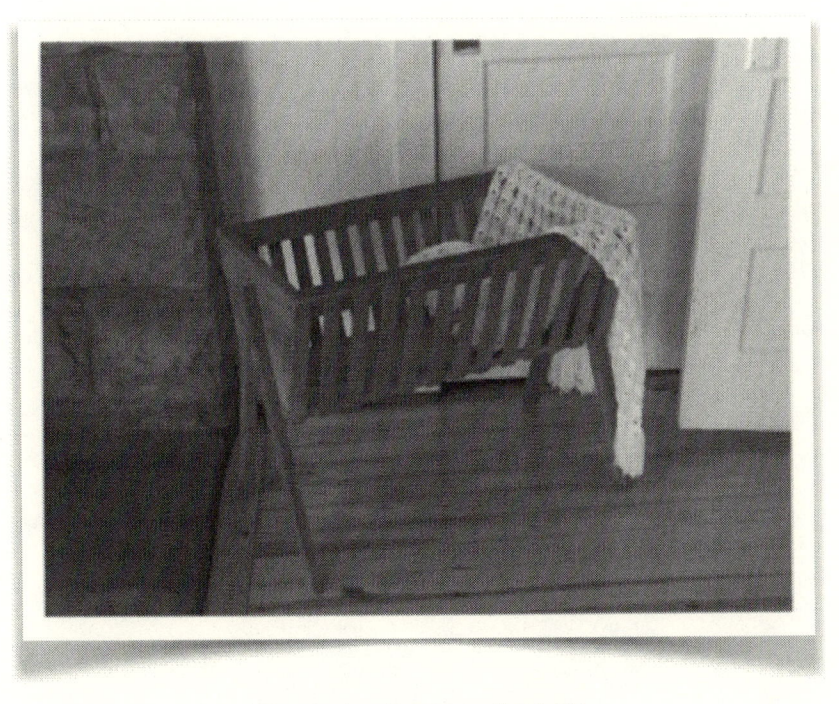

Photo by Amy Pennington Brudnicki

81

EXPOSED BEAM CEILING
THE BIG HOUSE

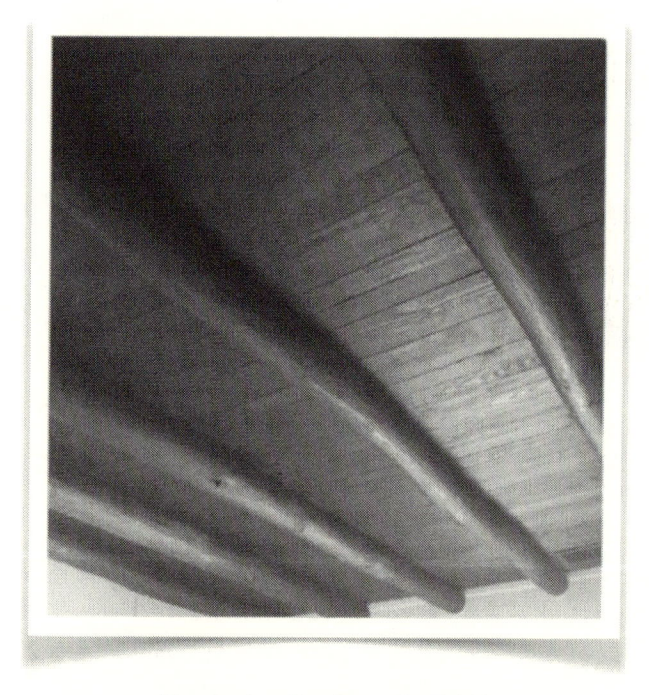

Photo by Amy Pennington Brudnicki

82

VINTAGE BOOKCASE IN MARY BRECKINRIDGE'S BEDROOM
THE BIG HOUSE

OCTOBER 17, 2015

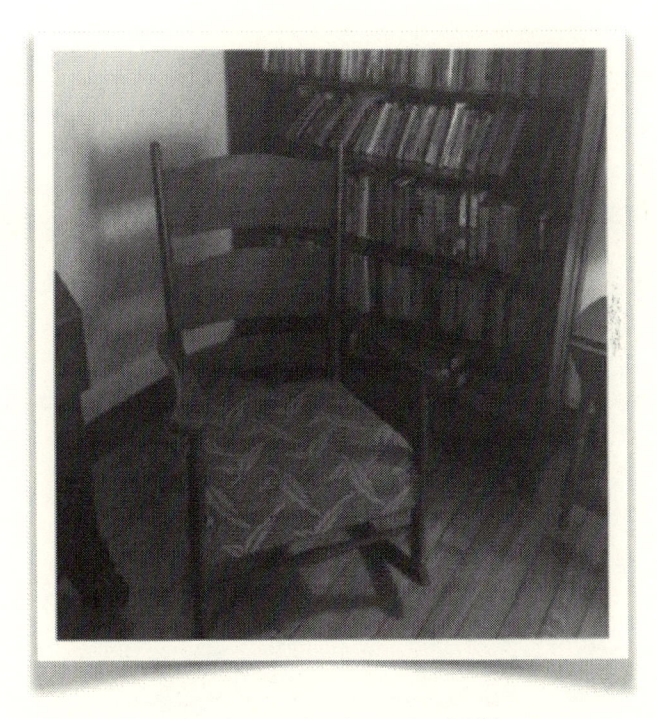

Photo by Amy Pennington Brudnicki

83

CONTINUING THE TRADITION
WENDOVER CHRISTMAS PLAY

HURRICANE CREEK COUSINS

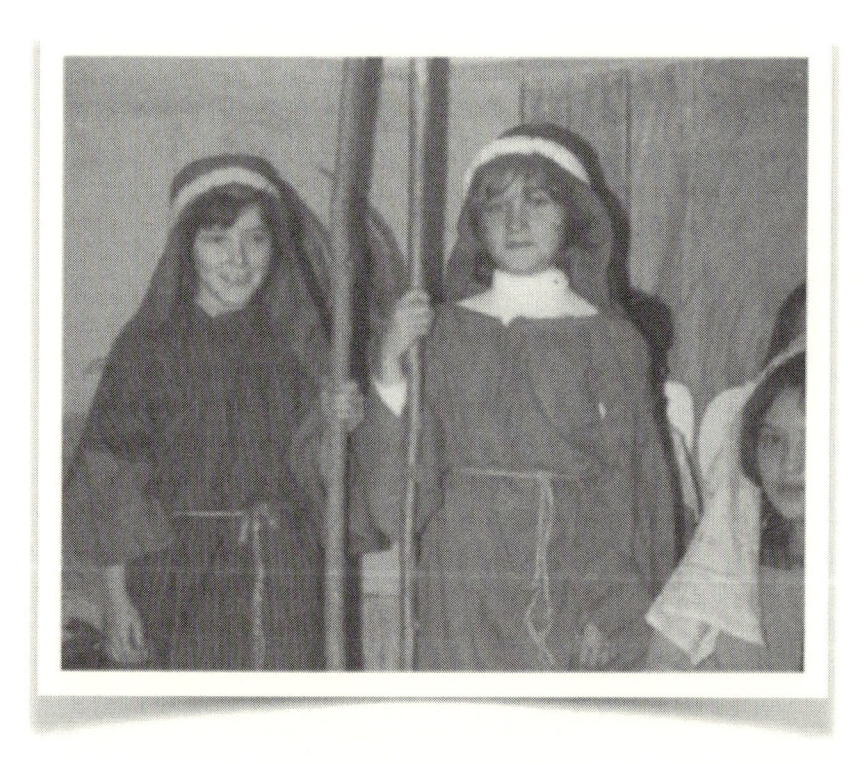

Missy Maggard & Tina McKinney

84

WENDOVER CHRISTMAS PLAY
THE GARDEN HOUSE

1975

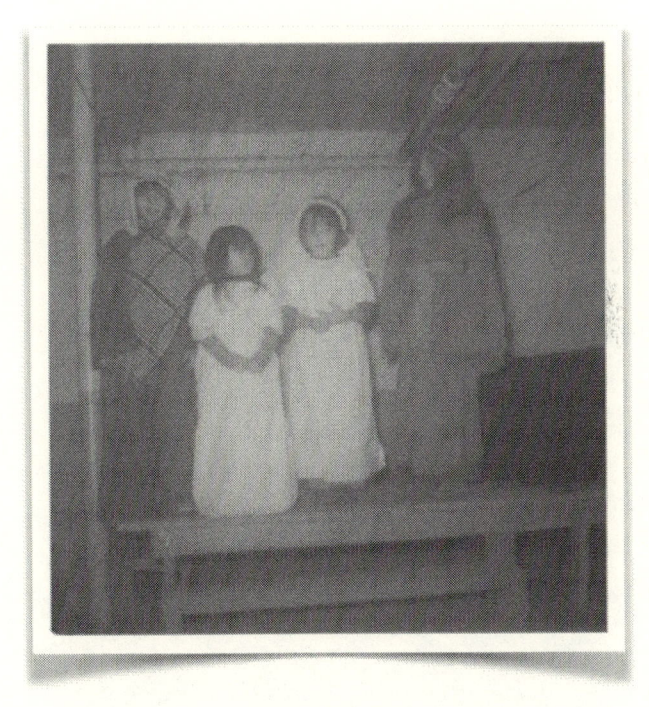

Lori McKinney, Tony Pennington, Kim Pennington, and Roger Howard

85

LITTLE ANGELS
WENDOVER CHRISTMAS PLAY
TINA MCKINNEY, MICHELLE CORNETT, AND AMY MAGGARD

Photo by Patricia McKinney

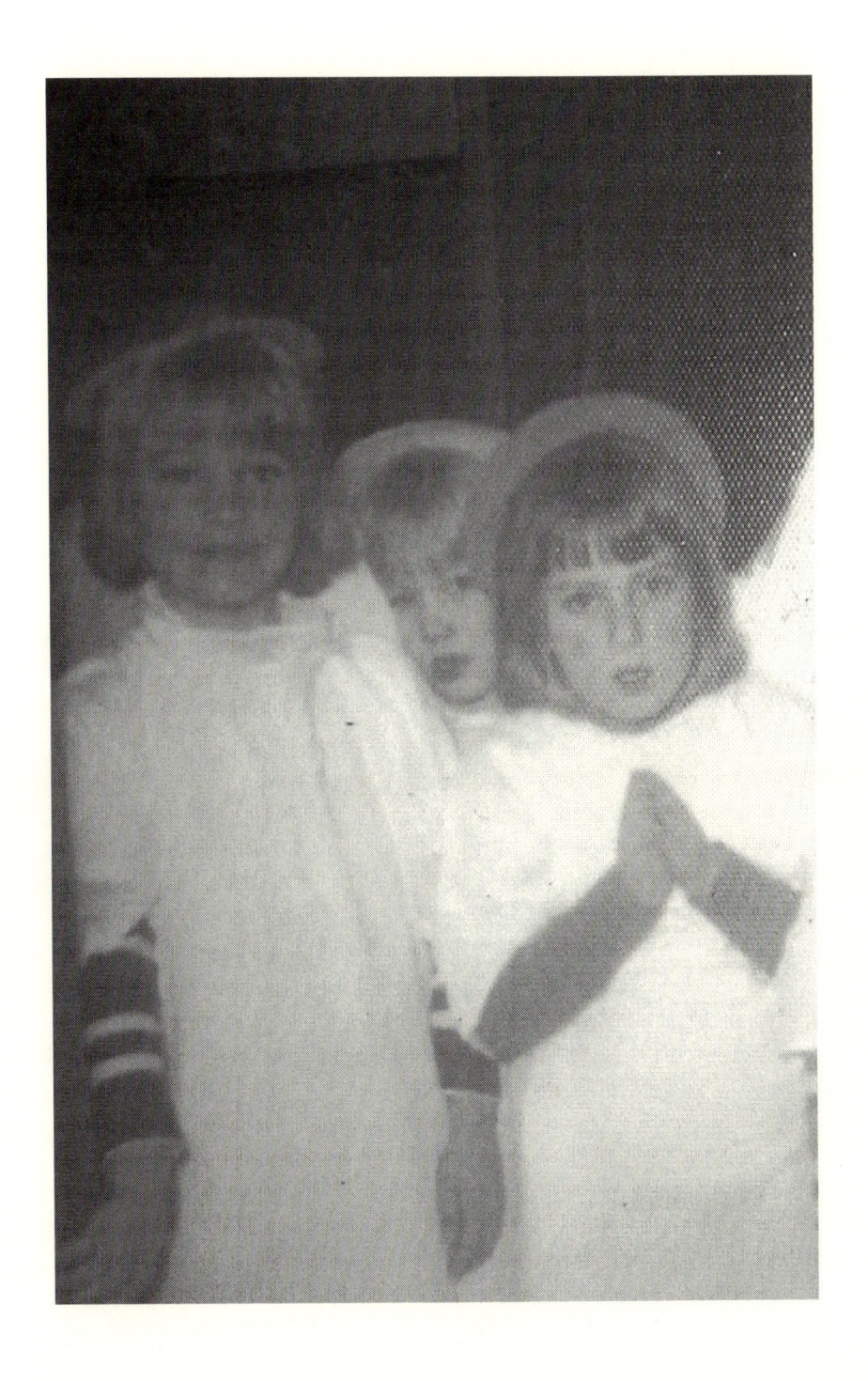

86

EXPLORERS

FIFTH GENERATION OF MAGGARDS TO EXPLORE THE HILLSIDE AT WENDOVER

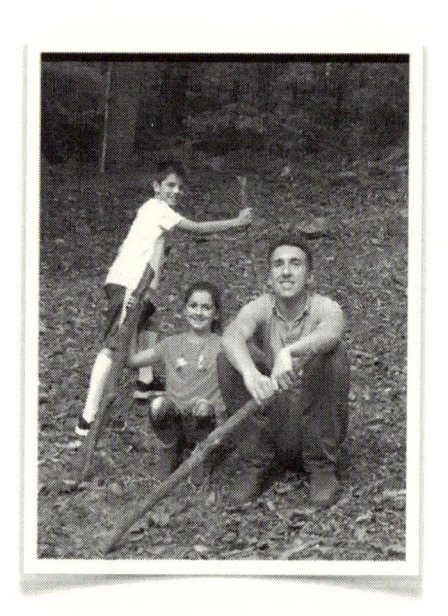

Photo by Amy Pennington Brudnicki

87

YOUNG EXPLORERS
FIFTH GENERATION OF MAGGARDS TO EXPLORE THE HILLSIDE AT WENDOVER

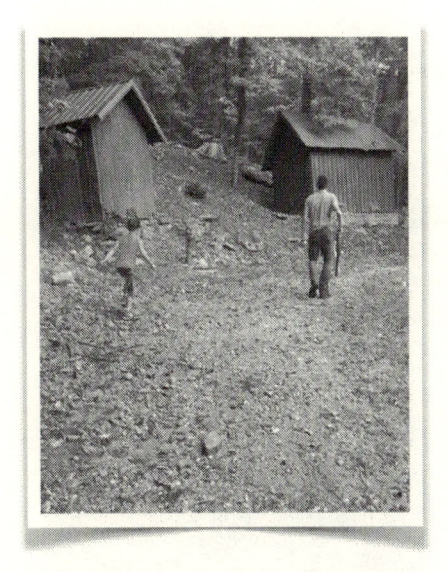

Photo by Amy Pennington Brudnicki

88

AMY PENNINGTON BRUDNICKI
HAGGIN NURSES DORM

LEGENDARY FLORENCE NIGHTINGALE BRICK FROM HER HOME. IT IS SAID THAT RUBBING THE BRICK BRINGS GOOD LUCK.

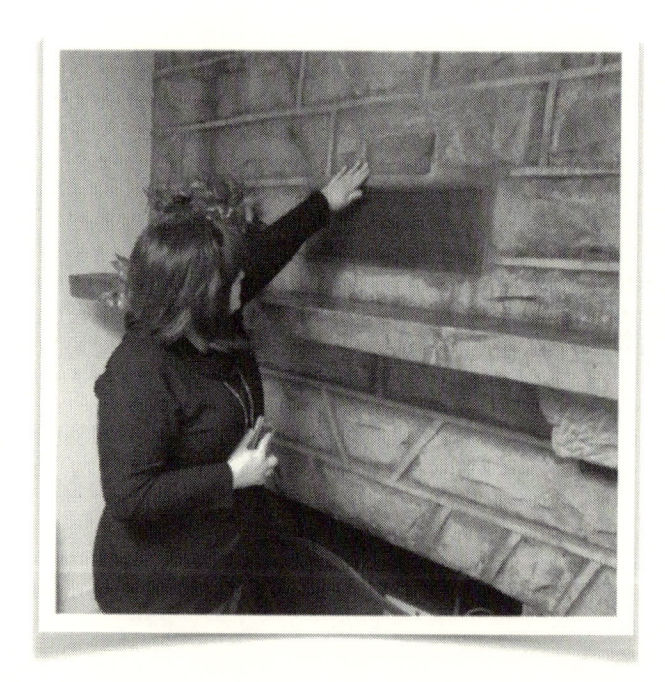

Photo by Michael Claussen

89

VINTAGE BOOKS
IN TWIN ROOM OF THE BIG HOUSE
OCTOBER 17, 2015

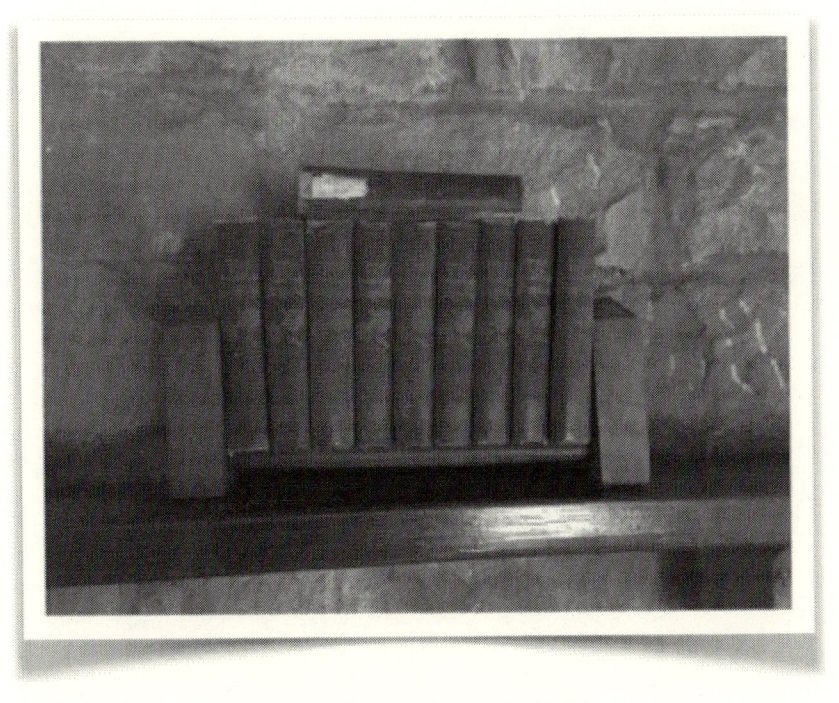

Photo by Amy Pennington Brudnicki

90

LUNCH WITH FRIENDS
THE BIG HOUSE
DECEMBER 2019

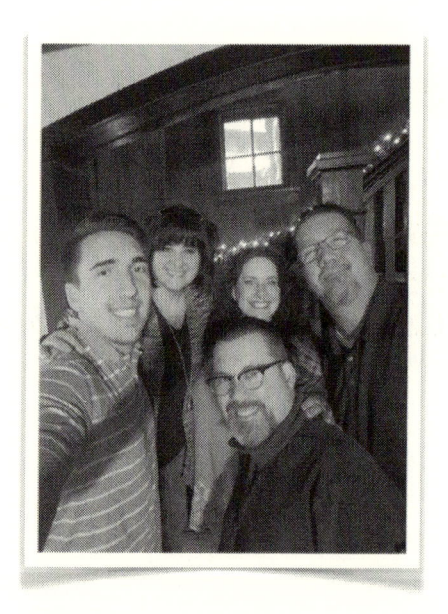

The Claussens & the Brudnicki's. Photo credit: Melody Claussen

91

VINTAGE FNS PHOTOS

The following pictures are vintage FNS photos, reprinted with permission from FNU.

" All photographs have been used with permission from Frontier Nursing University. For information on the use of these or other historic photographs please contact FNU@frontier.edu or 859-251-4700."

92

MARY BRECKINRIDGE
FOUNDER OF
THE FRONTIER NURSING SERVICE

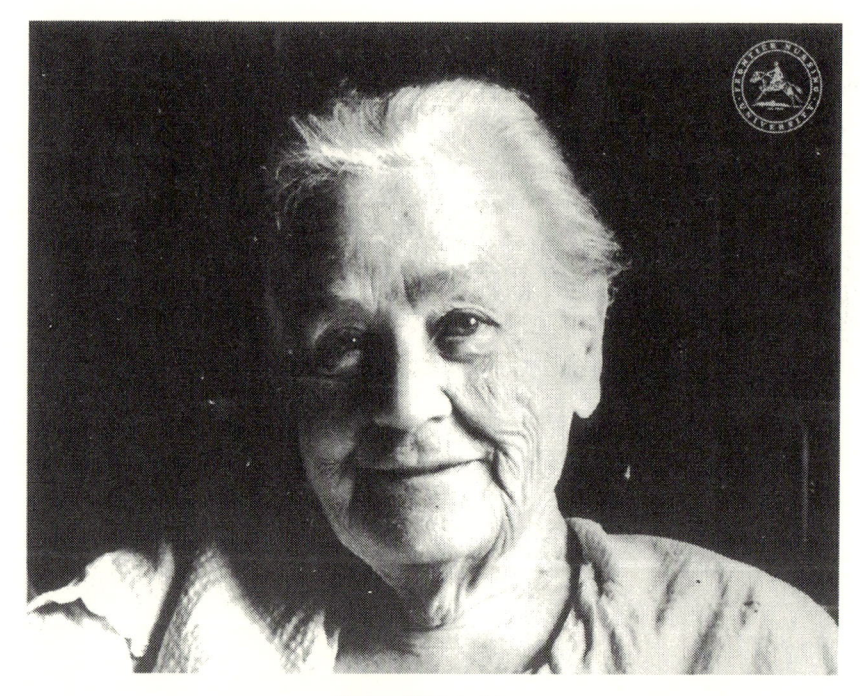

Source: FNU Archives

93

FRONTIER NURSING SERVICE
NURSES ON HORSEBACK

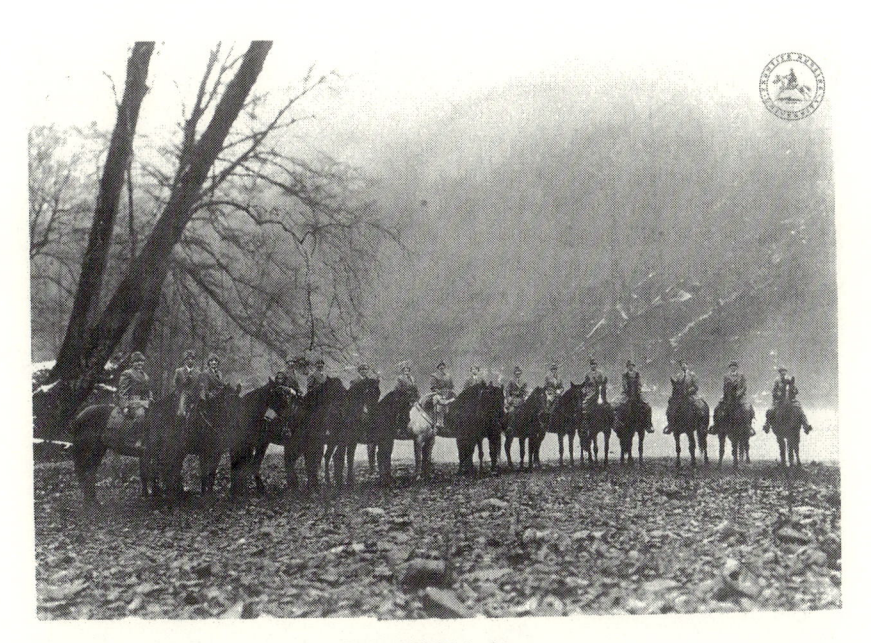

Source: FNU Archives

THE BIG HOUSE
MARY BRECKINRIDGE
& HELEN BROWNE

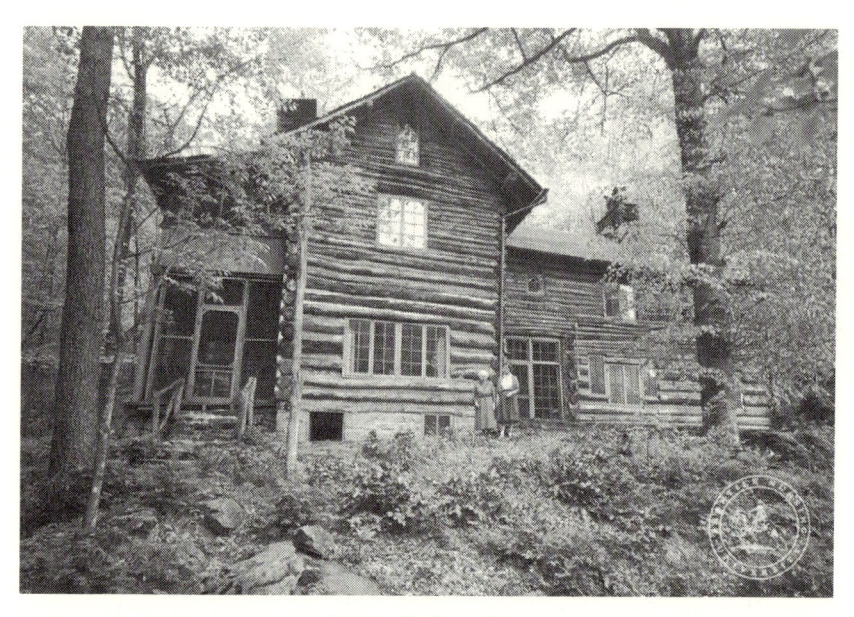

Source: FNU Archives

95

THE OLD HYDEN HOSPITAL
ON HOSPITAL HILL

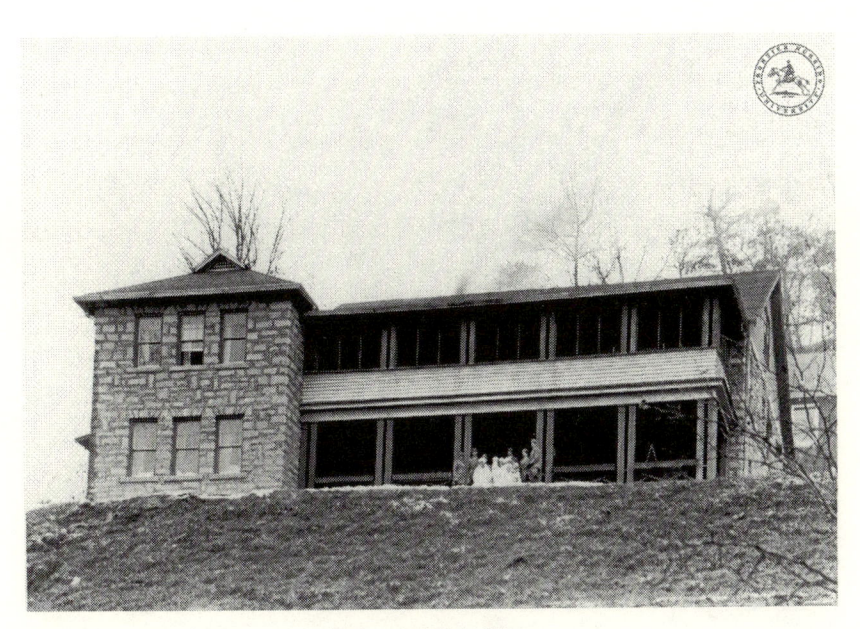

Source: FNU Archives

96

CHRISTMAS DINNER WITH THE COURIERS, 1928
THE BIG HOUSE'S DOG TROT DINING ROOM

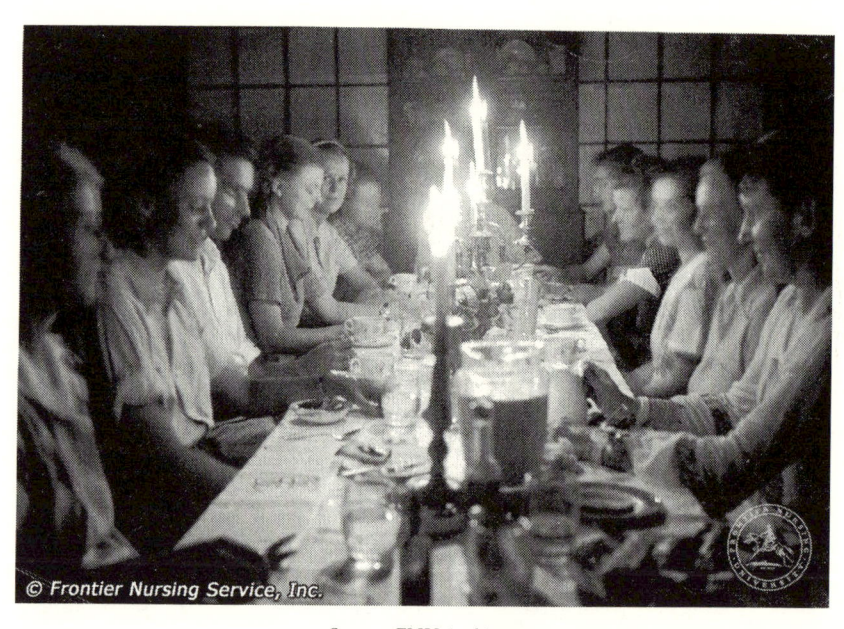

Source: FNU Archives

97

MARY BRECKINRIDGE
AND HER BELOVED ANIMALS

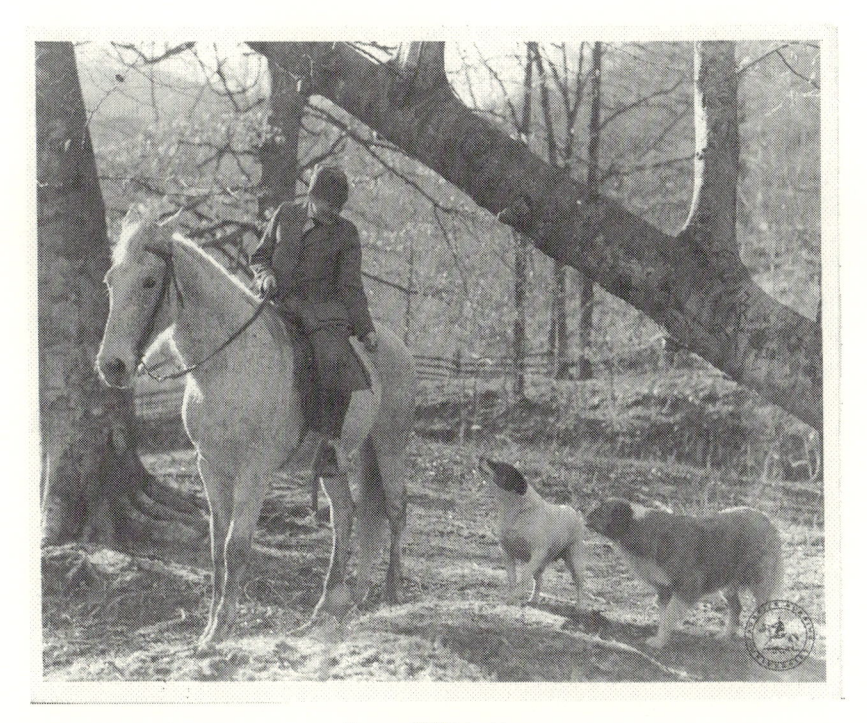

Source: FNU Archives

98

THE ORIGINAL GARDEN HOUSE

BUILT 1931

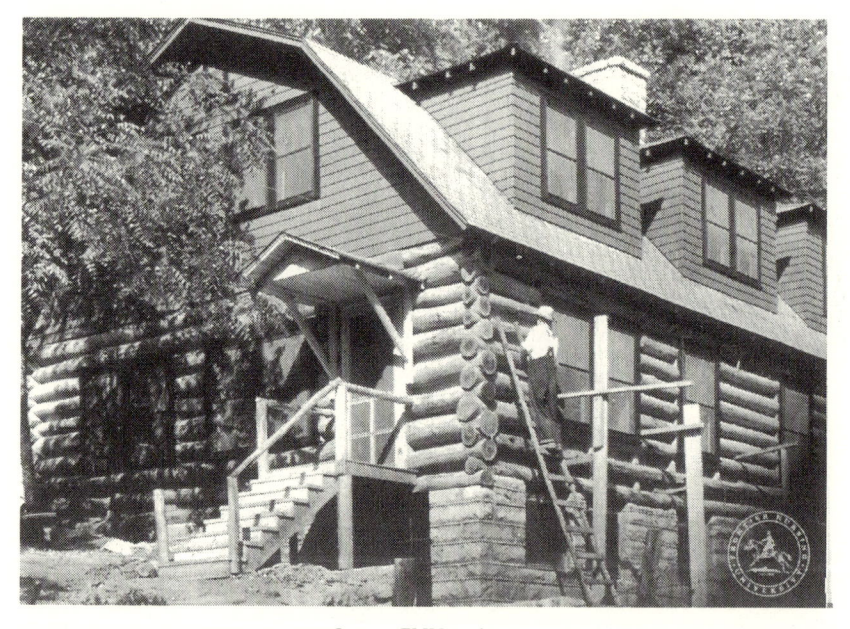

Source: FNU Archives

99

THE ORIGINAL GARDEN HOUSE
DESTROYED BY FIRE, 1942

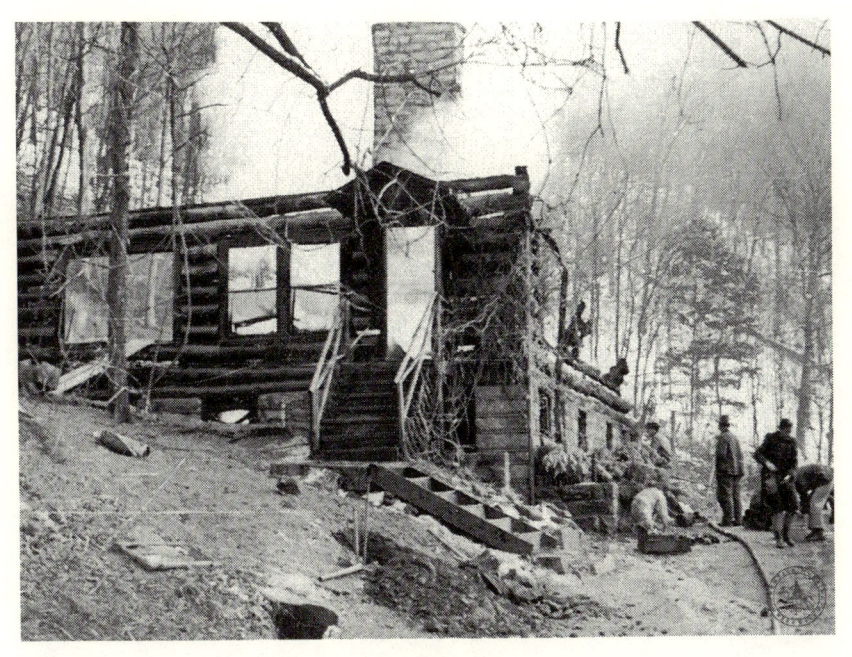

Source: FNU Archives

100

TRANSPORTATION, OLD VS. NEW
ANNE CUNDLE ON HORSEBACK
BETTY LESTER IN JEEP

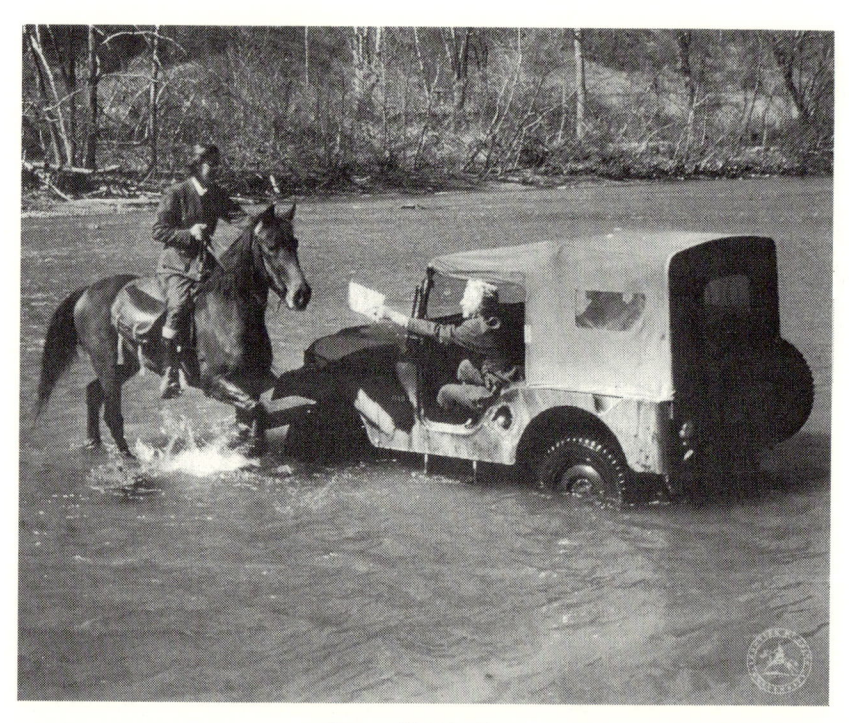

Source: FNU Archives

101

BETTY LESTER
AT OLD HYDEN HOSPITAL
HOSPITAL HILL

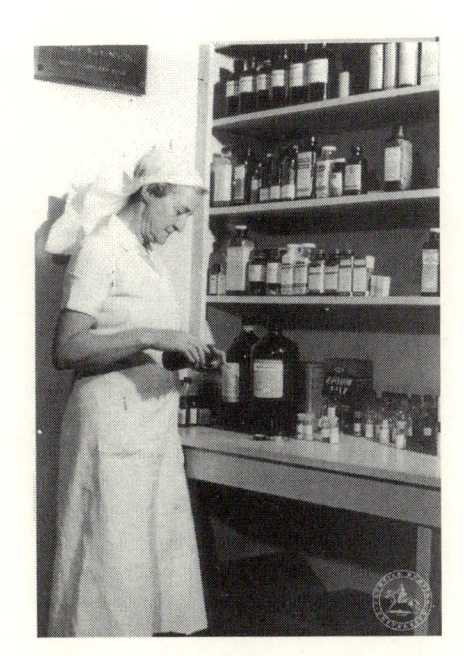

Source: FNU Archives

102

THE WENDOVER CABIN
SNOWY WONDERLAND

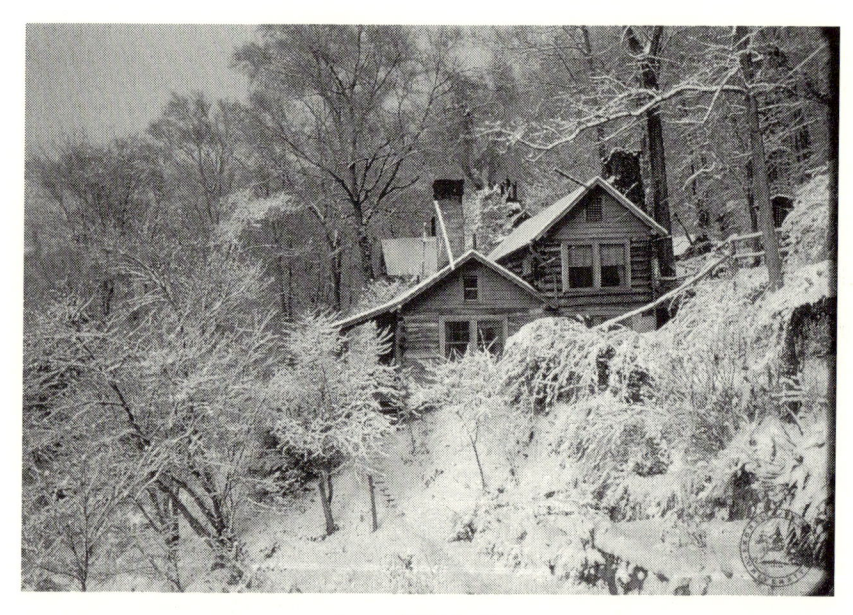

Source: FNU Archives

103

THE SADDLEBAG BABY

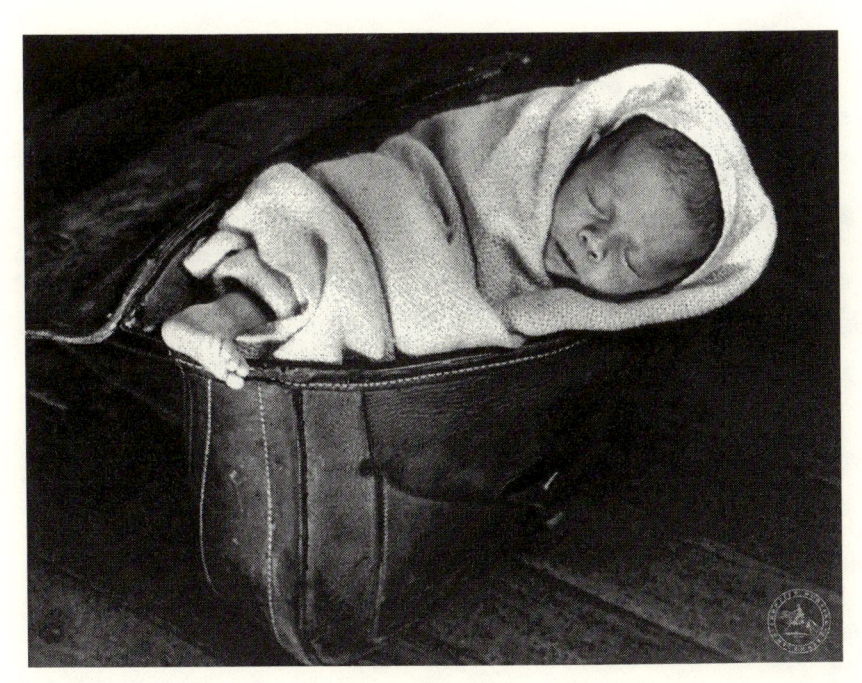

Source: FNU Archives

104

FNS NURSES
IN SUMMER RIDING UNIFORMS

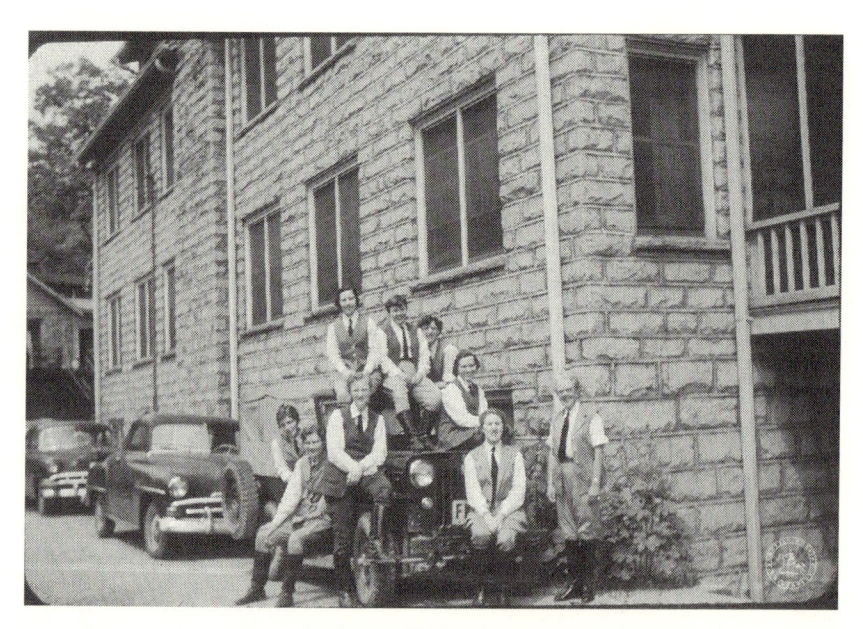

Source: FNU Archives

105

MARY BRECKINRIDGE
IN FNS WINTER RIDING UNIFORM

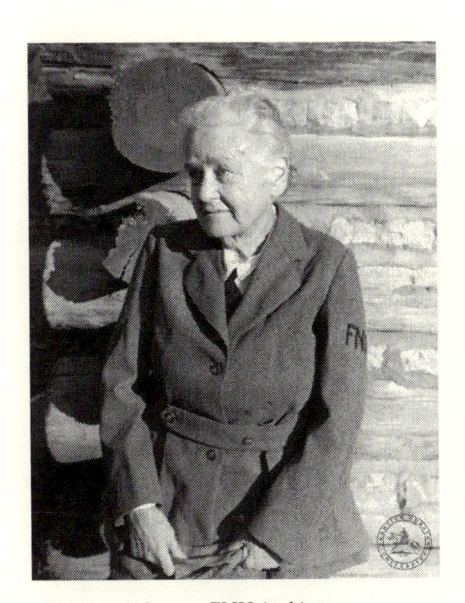

Source: FNU Archives

106

MARY BRECKINRIDGE
AND ONE OF HER FAVORITE HORSES, BABBETTE

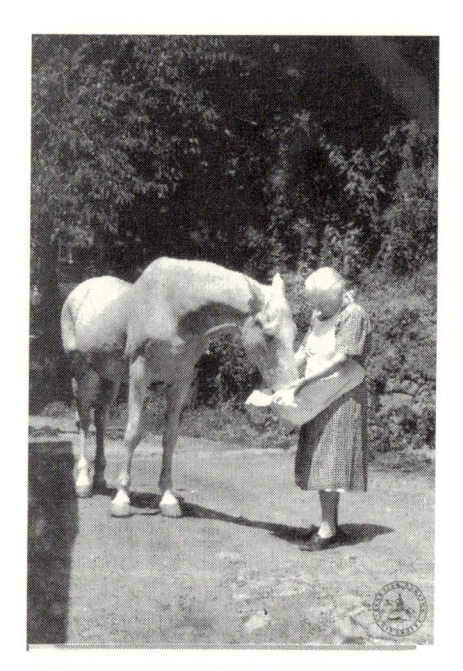

Source: FNU Archives

107

COURIERS WASHING THE JEEP
IN THE MIDDLE FORK RIVER

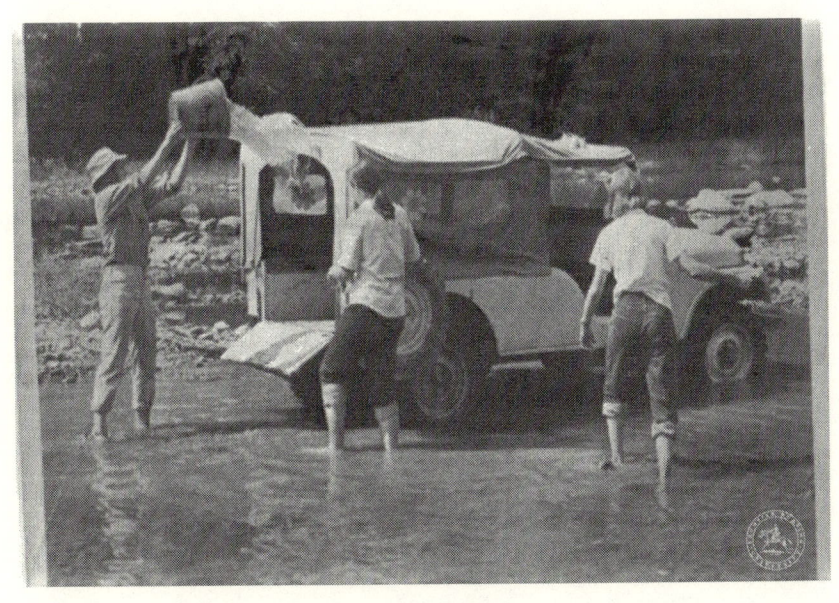

Source: FNU Archives

108

MARY BRECKINRIDGE
AND TEDDY BEAR, HER FIRST FRONTIER NURSING SERVICE HORSE

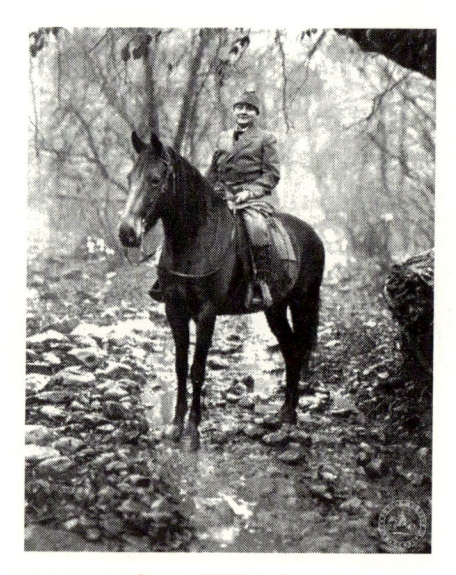

Source: FNU Archives

109

THE WENDOVER BARN

1955

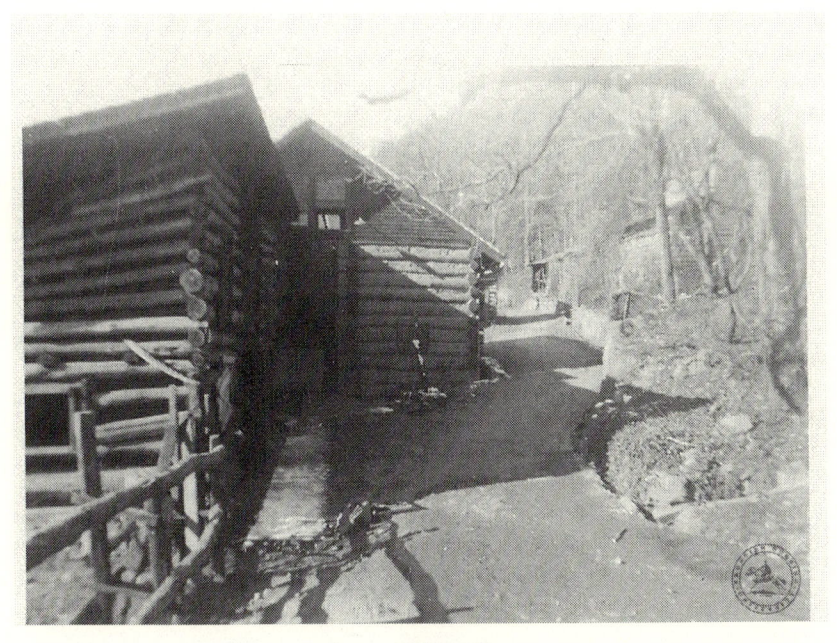

Source: FNU Archives

110

HOME DELIVERY

THE WALLS ARE COVERED WITH NEWSPAPER, SOMETHING THAT WAS COMMON IN MOUNTAIN HOMES.

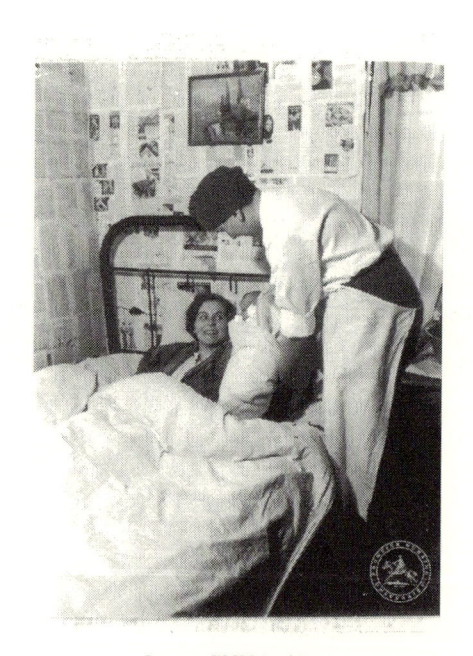

Source: FNU Archives

111

DAYS GONE BY
OLD HYDEN COURTHOUSE

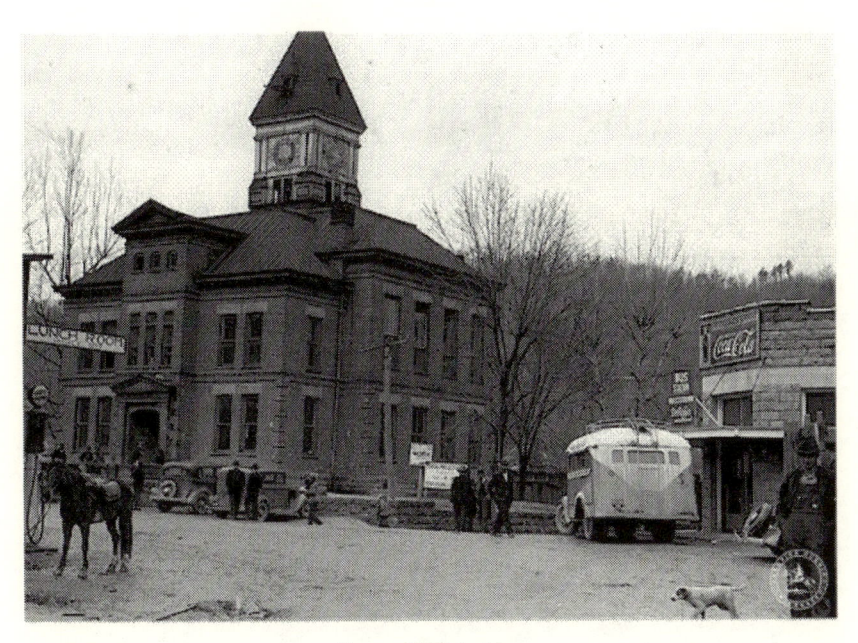

Source: FNU Archives

112

COURIERS ON HORSEBACK

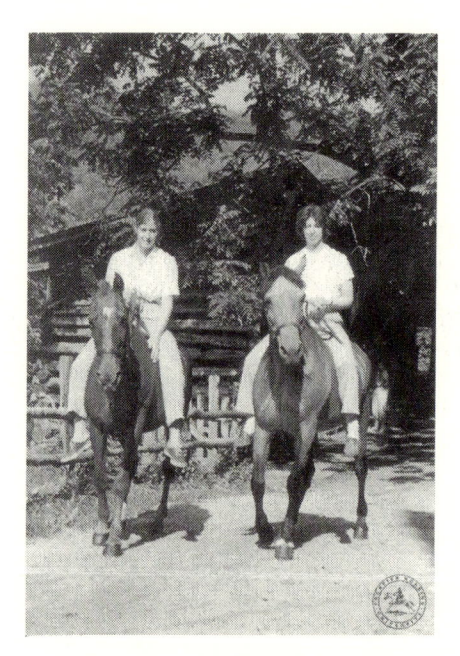

Source: FNU Archives

113

COURIER IN JEEP

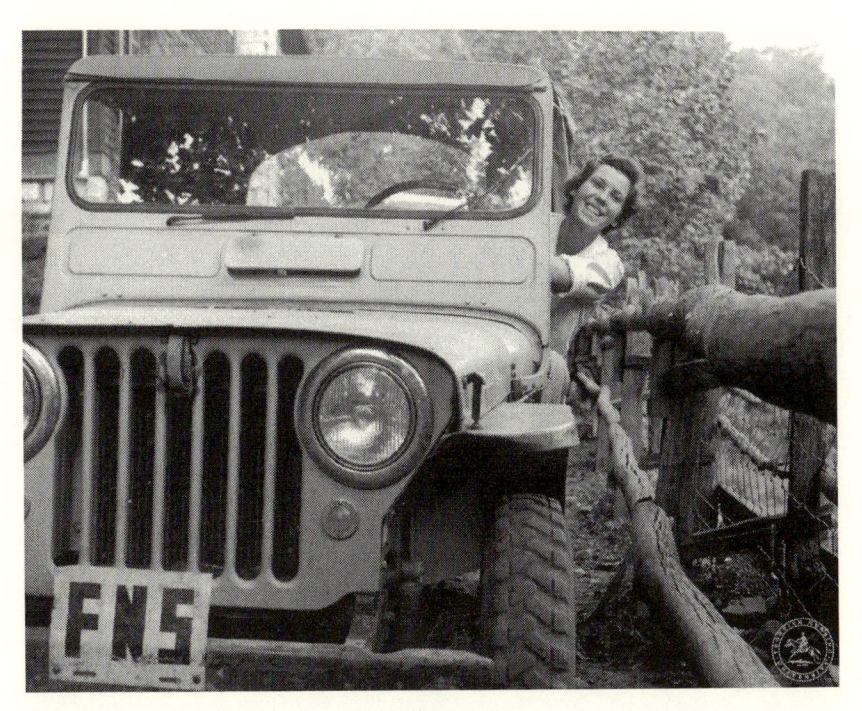

Source: FNU Archives

114

THE ORIGINAL WENDOVER BARN

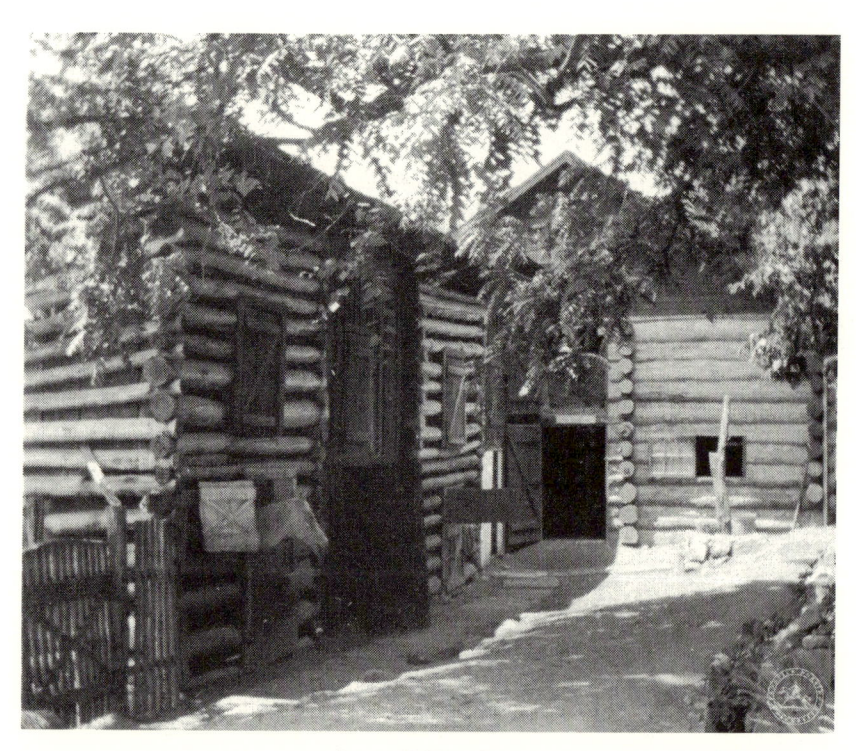

Source: FNU Archives

115

CHRISTMAS NATIVITY PLAY

AUTUMN 1962

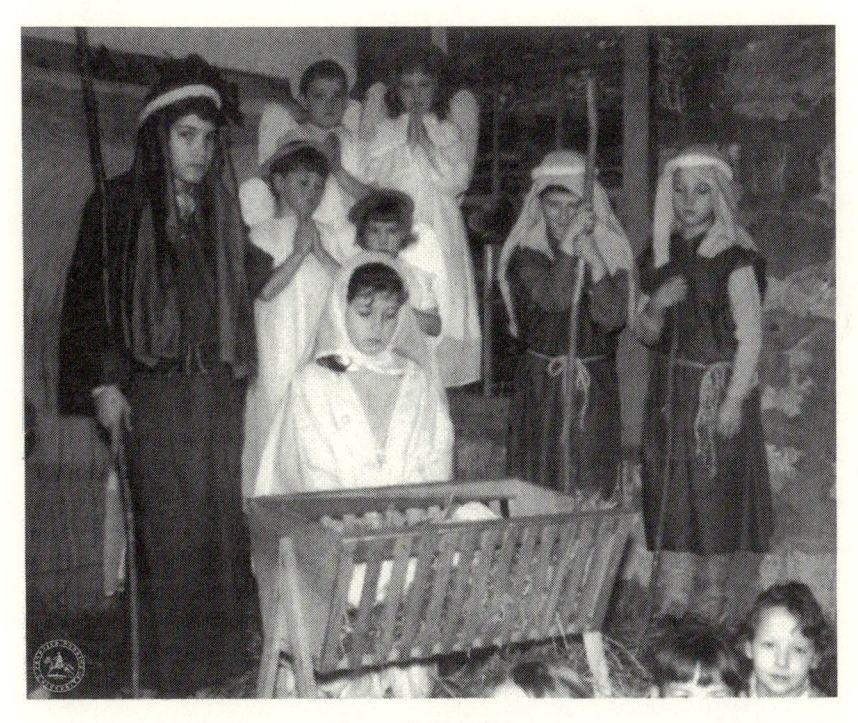

Source: FNU Archives

116

THE WENDOVER CABIN

ALSO REFERRED TO AS THE LOG CHAPEL. IT WAS LOCATED BETWEEN THE BARN AND THE BIG HOUSE.

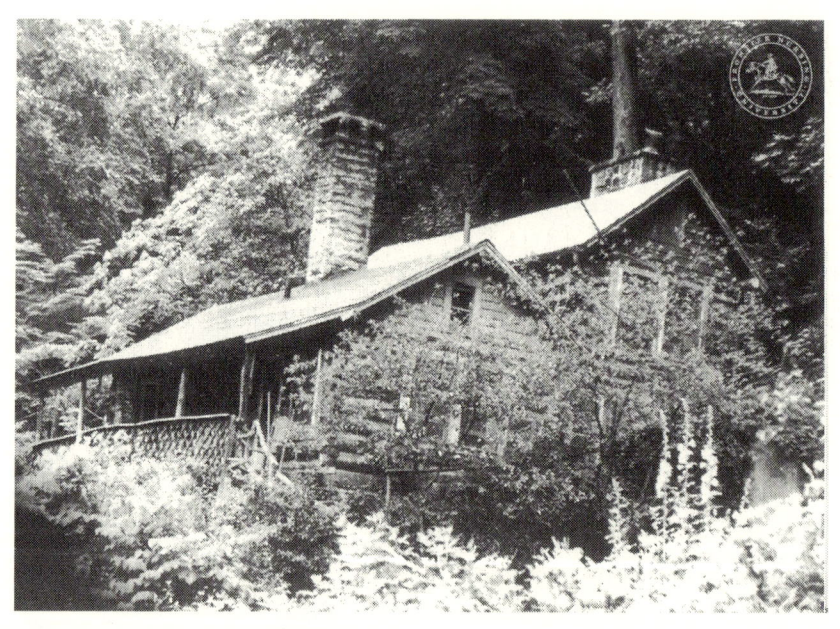

Source: FNU Archives

117

LOG CABIN CHAPEL
CHAPEL INSIDE THE WENDOVER CABIN

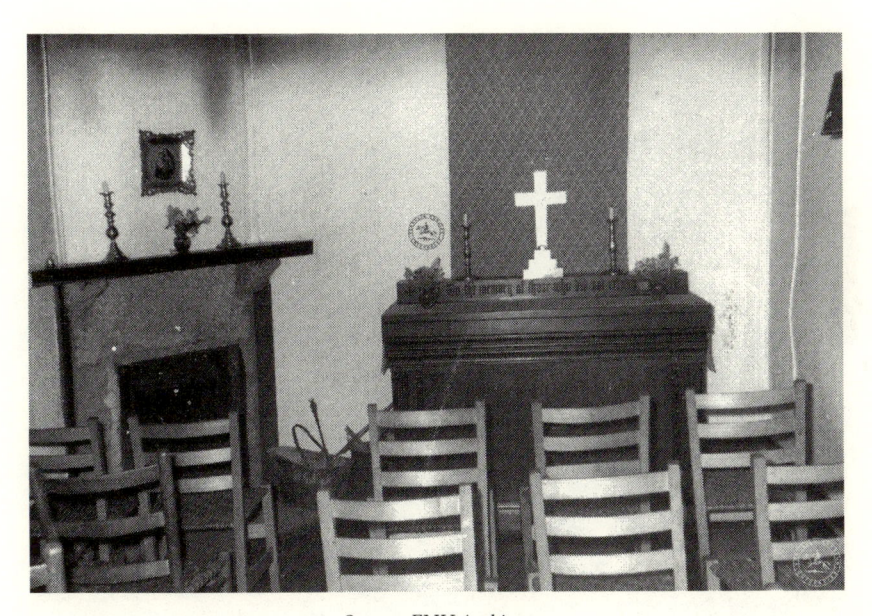

Source: FNU Archives

118

PIG ALLEY

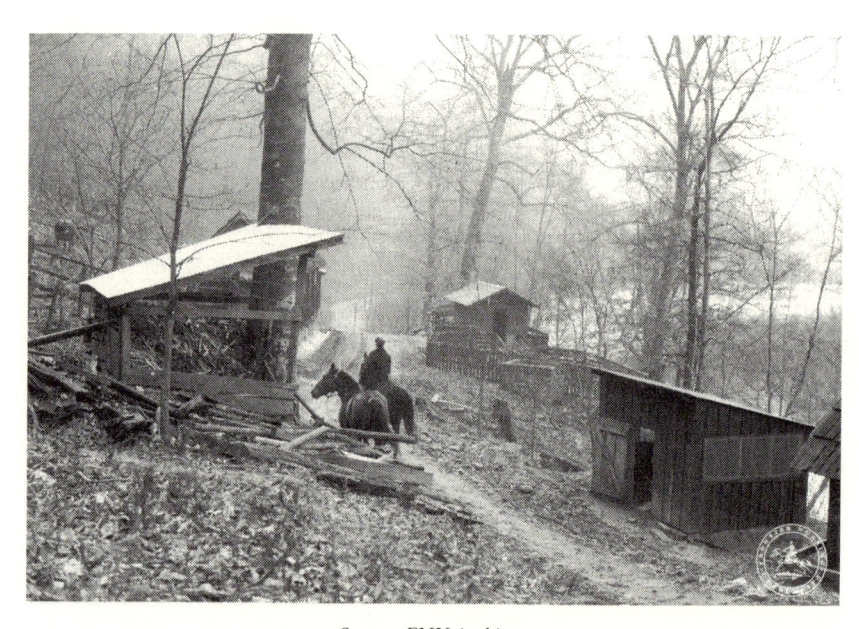

Source: FNU Archives

119

NURSES ON HORSEBACK

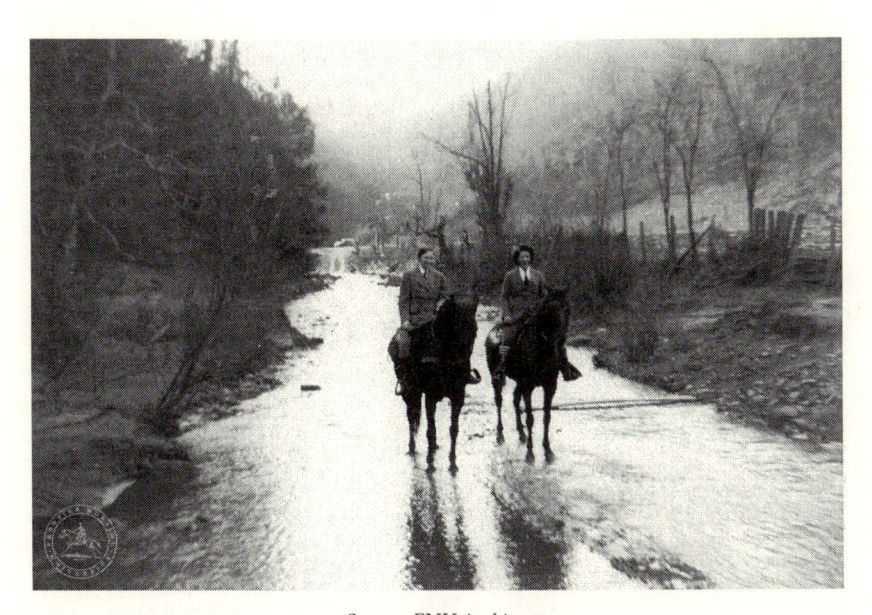

Source: FNU Archives

120

A YOUNG MARY BRECKINRIDGE

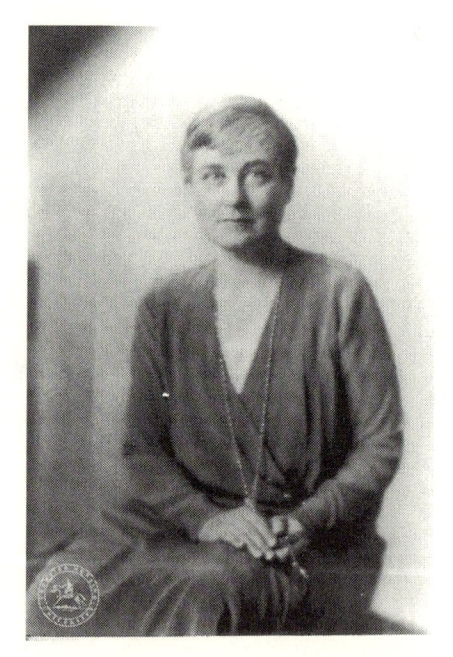

Source: FNU Archives

121

QUARTERLY BULLETIN PHOTOS

THE FOLLOWING PICTURES are vintage FNS photos, reprinted with permission from FNU from their Frontier Nursing Service Quarterly Bulletins.

" ALL PHOTOGRAPHS HAVE BEEN USED with permission from Frontier Nursing University. For information on the use of these or other historic photographs please contact FNU@frontier.edu or 859-251-4700 ."

FIRST QUARTERLY BULLETIN
SOURCE: FNU ARCHIVES

THE KENTUCKY COMMITTEE FOR MOTHERS AND BABIES, PREDECESSOR TO FNS

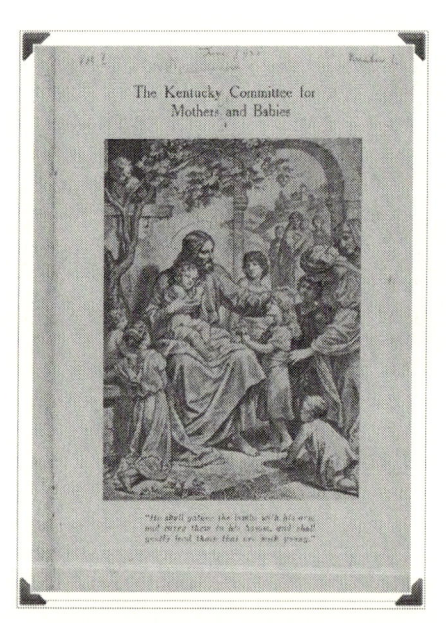

June 1925 FNS Quarterly Bulletin (14A)

123

CHILDREN'S OUTDOOR WARD
SOURCE: FNU ARCHIVES

THE QUARTERLY BULLETIN OF THE FRONTIER NURSING SERVICE, INC.

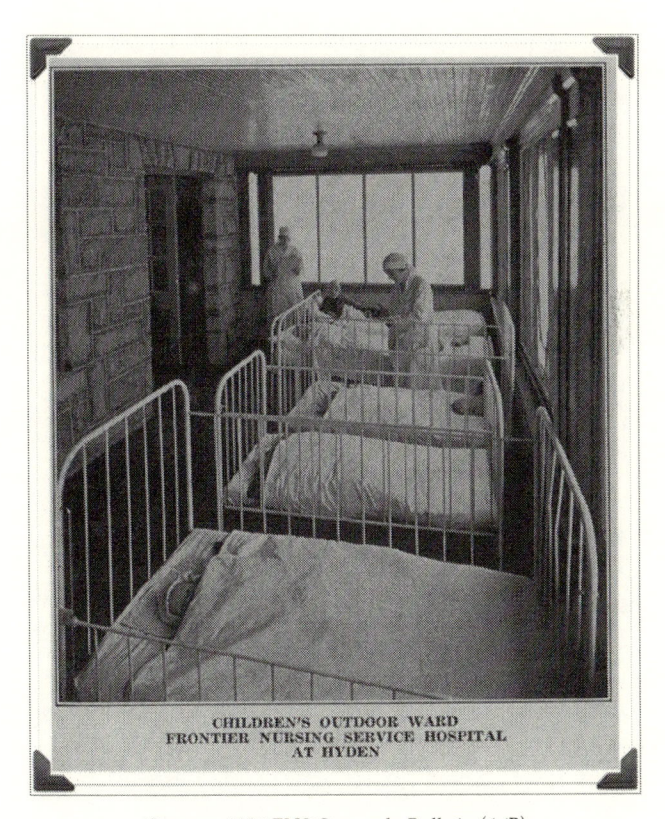

Summer 1931 FNS Quarterly Bulletin (14B)

124

FLOATING LOGS DOWN THE MIDDLE FORK

SOURCE: FNU ARCHIVES

THE QUARTERLY BULLETIN OF THE FRONTIER NURSING SERVICE, INC.

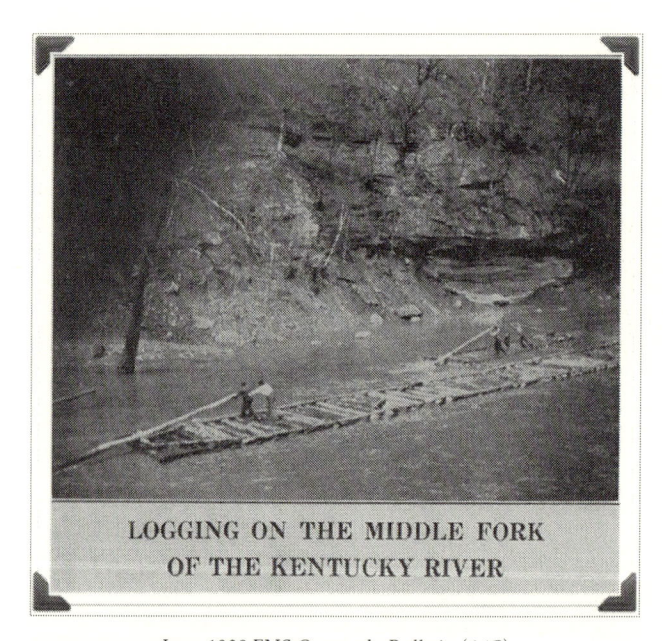

LOGGING ON THE MIDDLE FORK
OF THE KENTUCKY RIVER

June 1929 FNS Quarterly Bulletin (14C)

125

BUILDING THE CHAPEL
SOURCE: FNU ARCHIVES

ST. CHRISTOPHER'S CHAPEL

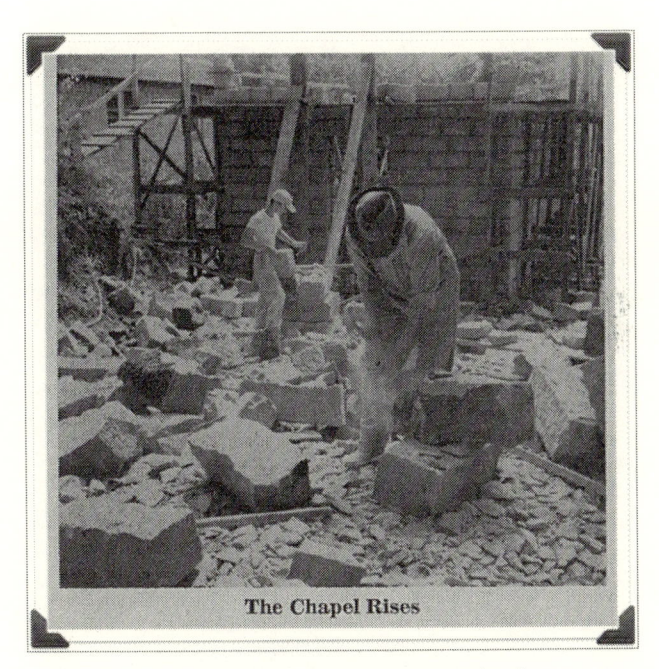

Summer 1960 FNS Quarterly Bulletin (14D)

126

CHAPEL CONSTRUCTION
SOURCE: FNU ARCHIVES

PHOTO BY MR. J.A. RIORDAN

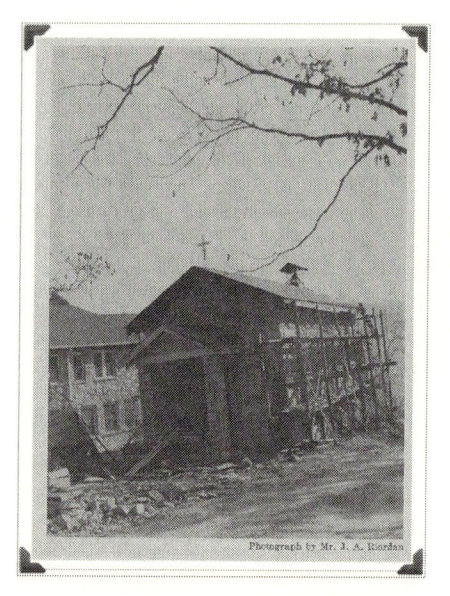

Autumn 1960 FNS Quarterly Bulletin (14E)

127

MOLLY LEE
SOURCE: FNU ARCHIVES

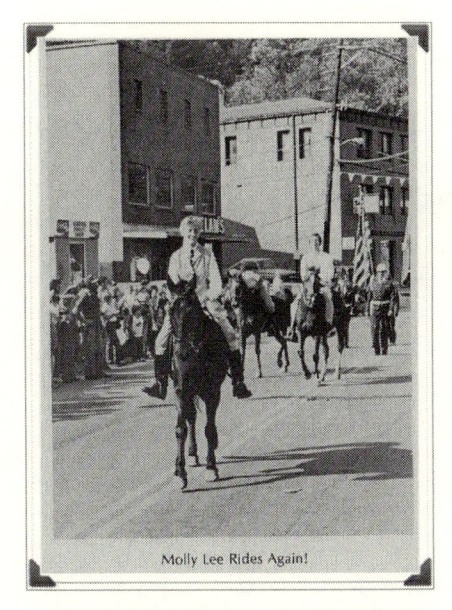

Molly Lee Rides Again!

Autumn 1982 FNS Quarterly Bulletin (14F)

128

ANNA MAY JANUARY
SOURCE: FNU ARCHIVES

BELOVED NURSE-MIDWIFE

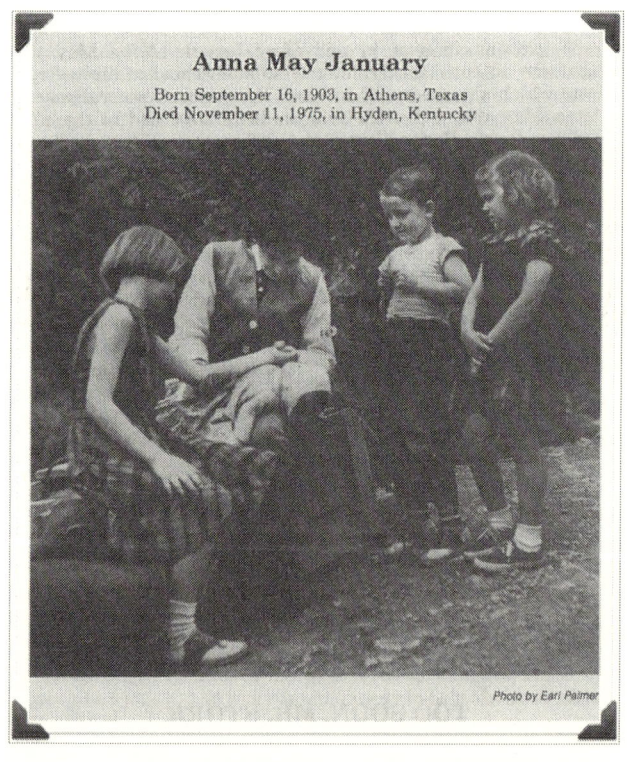

Anna May January
Born September 16, 1903, in Athens, Texas
Died November 11, 1975, in Hyden, Kentucky

Photo by Earl Palmer

Autumn 1975 FNS Quarterly Bulletin (14G)

CHRISTMAS PAGEANT
SOURCE: FNU ARCHIVES
PHOTO BY ANNE CUNDLE

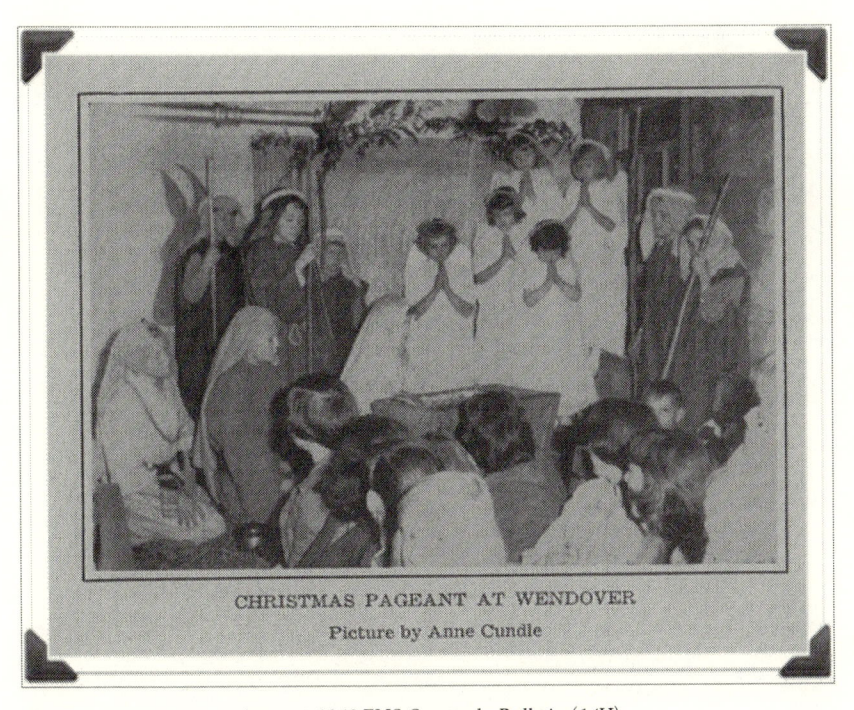

Autumn 1960 FNS Quarterly Bulletin (14H)

130

A BABY A DAY
SOURCE: FNU ARCHIVES

SPRING 1931 FNS QUARTERLY BULLETIN
(14I & 14J)

"A BABY A DAY is about our record now. Each cost his parents $5. That fee covers delivery, pre-natal and postpartum care. If they have no cash, and they rarely have, the fee may be paid in kind or in labor—skins of varmints, fodder for the horses, split-bottom chairs, or quilted "kivver". In the last two years Frontier Nurses delivered 583 mothers in childbirth without one maternal death. 101 in the last three months." [3X]

IN THE TRADITIONAL MOUNTAIN BIRTH, THE NURSE IS SUMMONED, AND THE FAMILY GATHERS 'ROUND, AWAITING THE ARRIVAL OF THE NEWEST ADDITION TO THE FAMILY.

A BABY A DAY

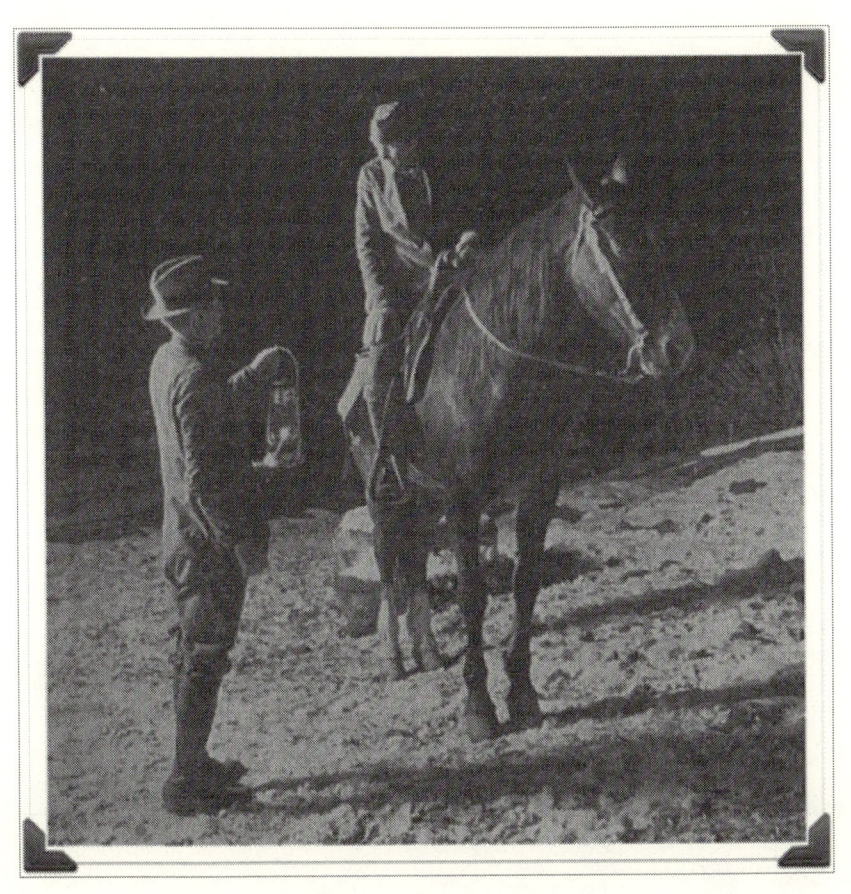

Spring 1931 FNS Quarterly Bulletin (I)

SPRING 1931 FNS QUARTERLY BULLETIN (14I & 14J)

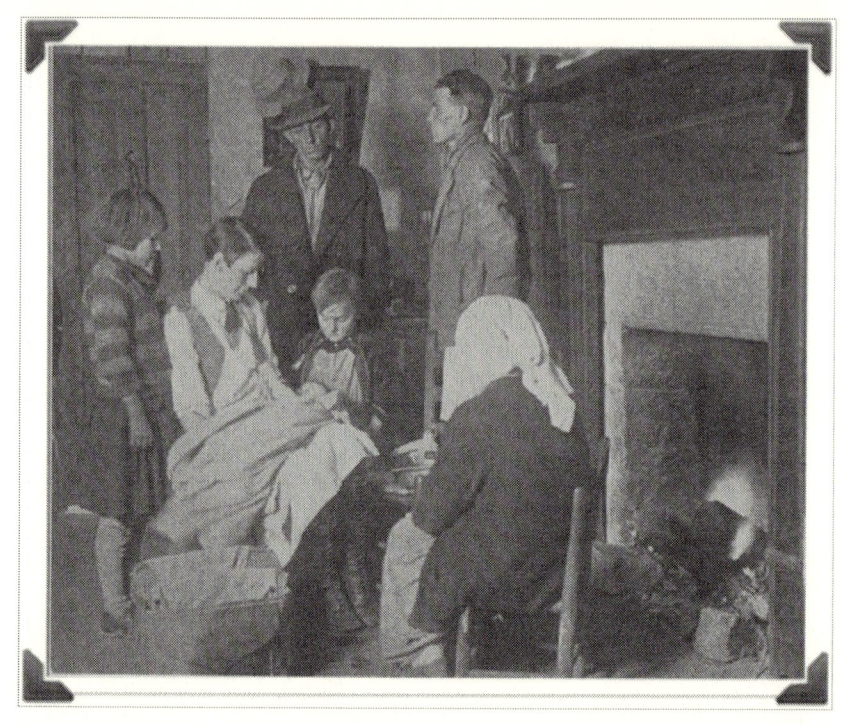

Spring 1931 FNS Quarterly Bulletin (J)

131

WENDOVER GEESE
SOURCE: FNU ARCHIVES

PHOTO BY HOUGHT BARBER

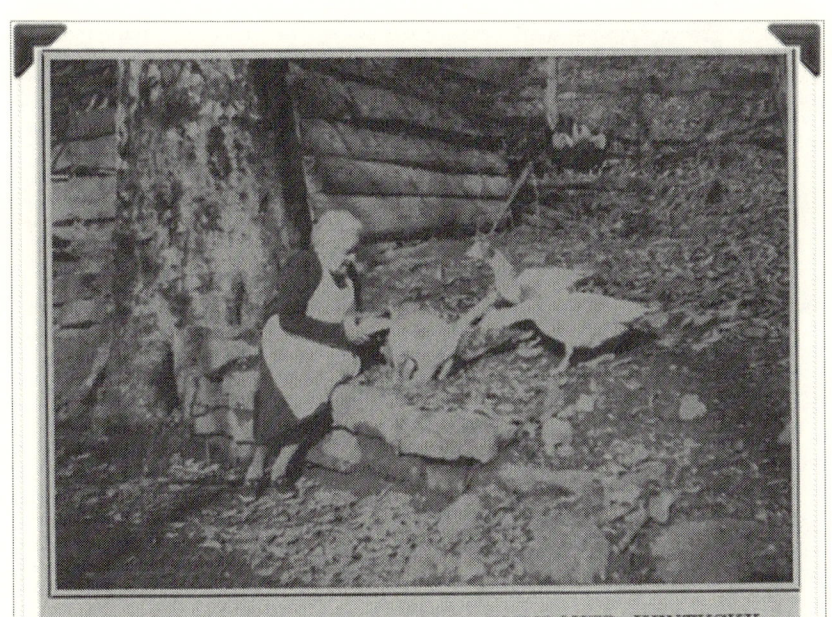

MARY BRECKINRIDGE (LEFT) AT WENDOVER, KENTUCKY
Taken just before she entered her 80th year by courier Hought Barber
Her friends are Tom, the yellow barn cat,
and Dilly (gander) and Dally (goose).

Spring 1960 FNS Quarterly Bulletin (14K)

132

HELEN BROWNE & ROGERS BEASLEY
SOURCE: FNU ARCHIVES
PHOTO BY GABRIELLE BEASLEY

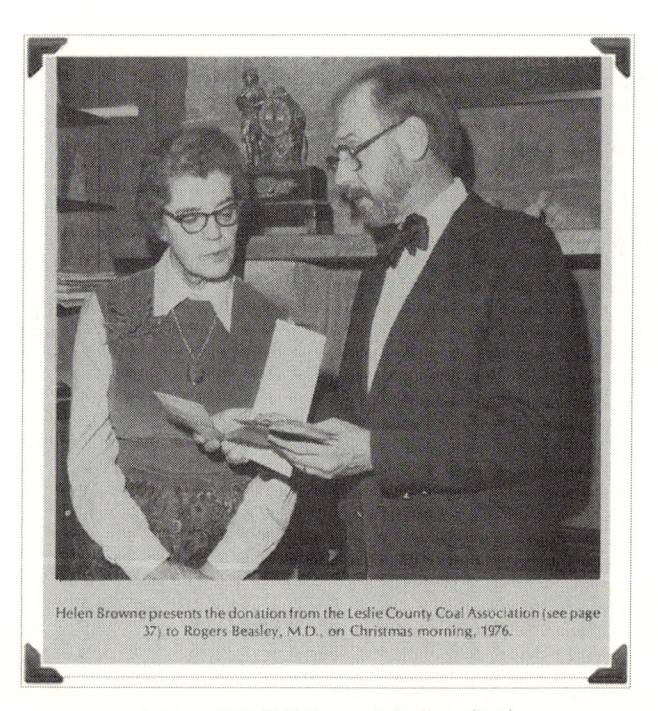

Helen Browne presents the donation from the Leslie County Coal Association (see page 37) to Rogers Beasley, M.D., on Christmas morning, 1976.

Autumn 1976 FNS Quarterly Bulletin (14L)

133

COURIER MARGO SQUIBB AS SANTA AND JACK BEGLEY
SOURCE: FNU ARCHIVES

PHOTO BY GABRIELLE BEASLEY

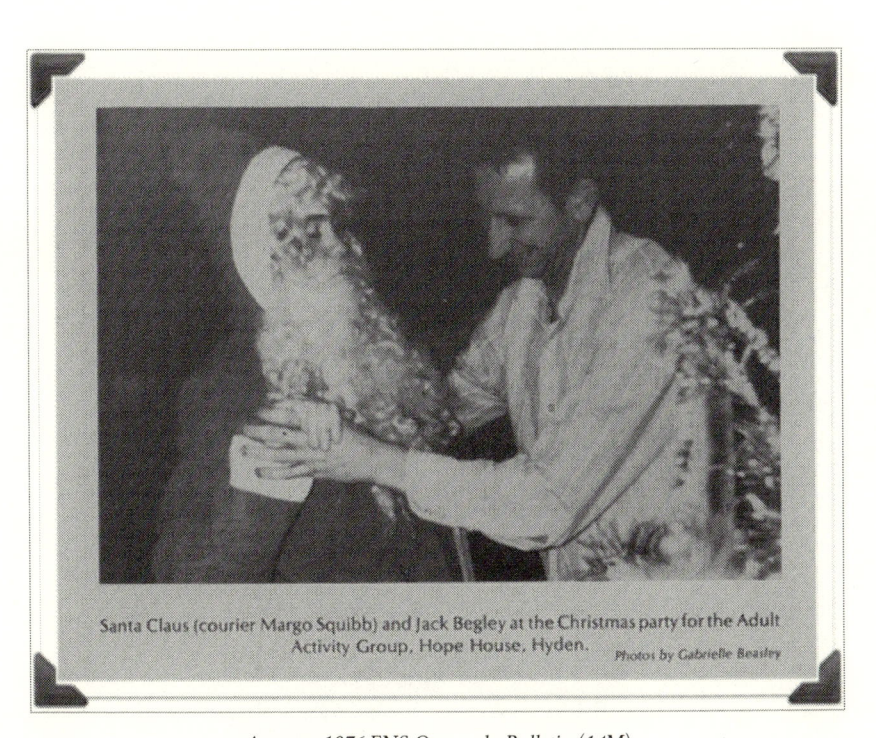

Santa Claus (courier Margo Squibb) and Jack Begley at the Christmas party for the Adult Activity Group, Hope House, Hyden. *Photo by Gabrielle Beasley*

Autumn 1976 FNS Quarterly Bulletin (14M)

134

FRONTIER NURSES
SOURCE: FNU ARCHIVES

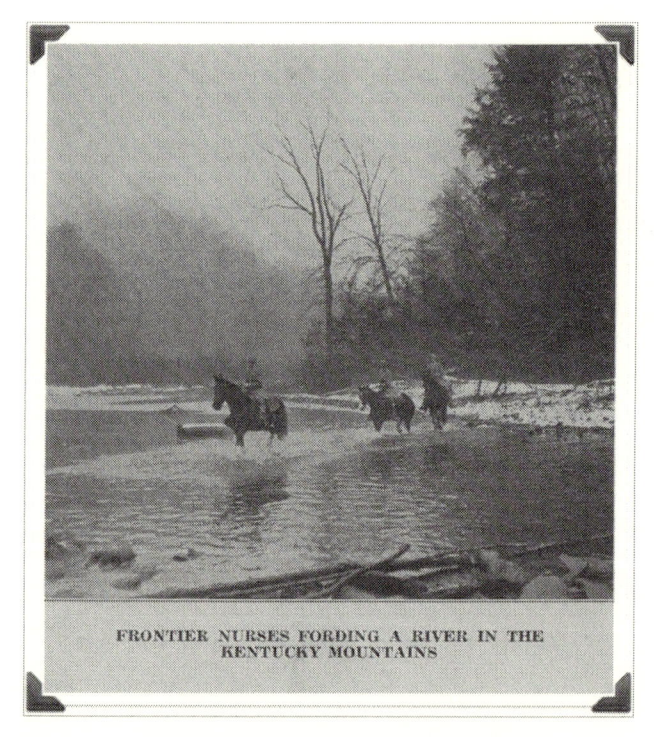

FRONTIER NURSES FORDING A RIVER IN THE
KENTUCKY MOUNTAINS

Winter 1931 FNS Quarterly Bulletin (14N)

135

CREEK CLINIC
SOURCE: FNU ARCHIVES

PHOTO BY TOAD HALL

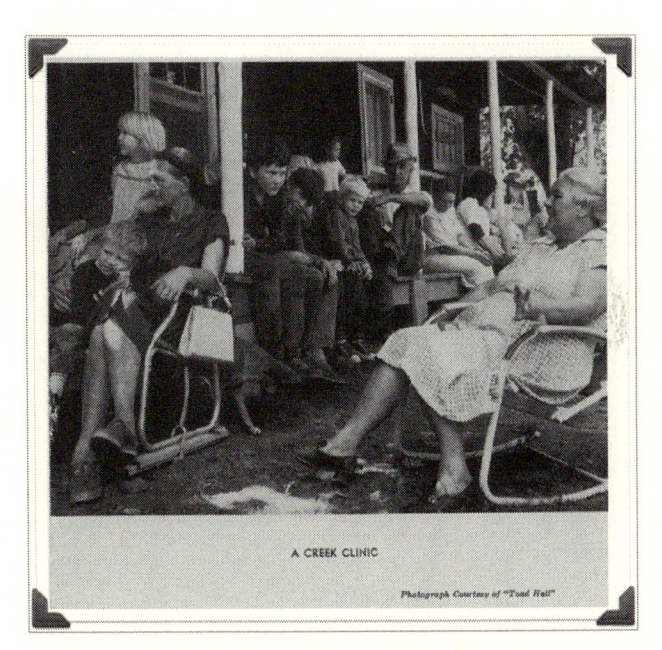

Summer 1974 FNS Quarterly Bulletin (140)

136

MARLENE WOOTON
SOURCE: FNU ARCHIVES

TEN THOUSANDTH FNS BABY

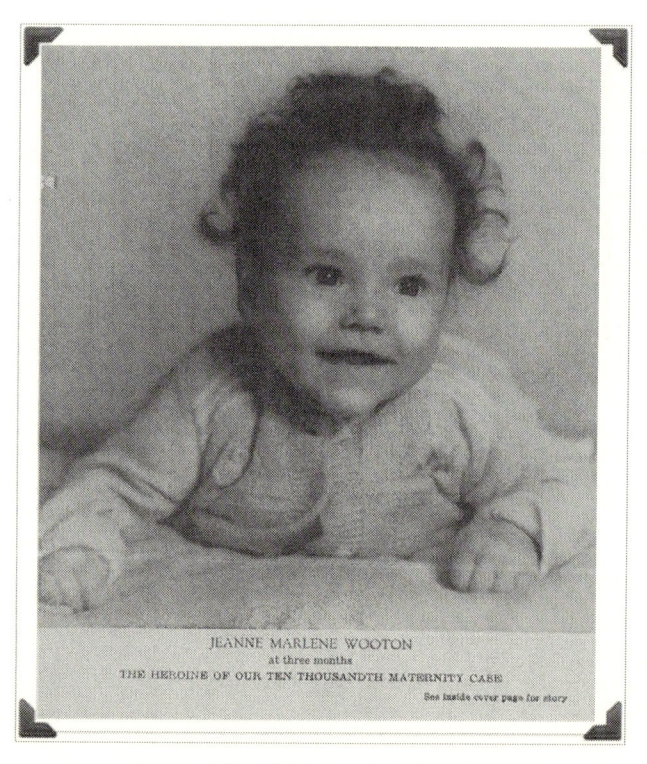

JEANNE MARLENE WOOTON
at three months
THE HEROINE OF OUR TEN THOUSANDTH MATERNITY CASE
See inside cover page for story

Autumn 1954 FNS Quarterly Bulletin (14P)

137

STEPS TO OLD HYDEN HOSPITAL
SOURCE: FNU ARCHIVES
PHOTO BY TOAD HALL

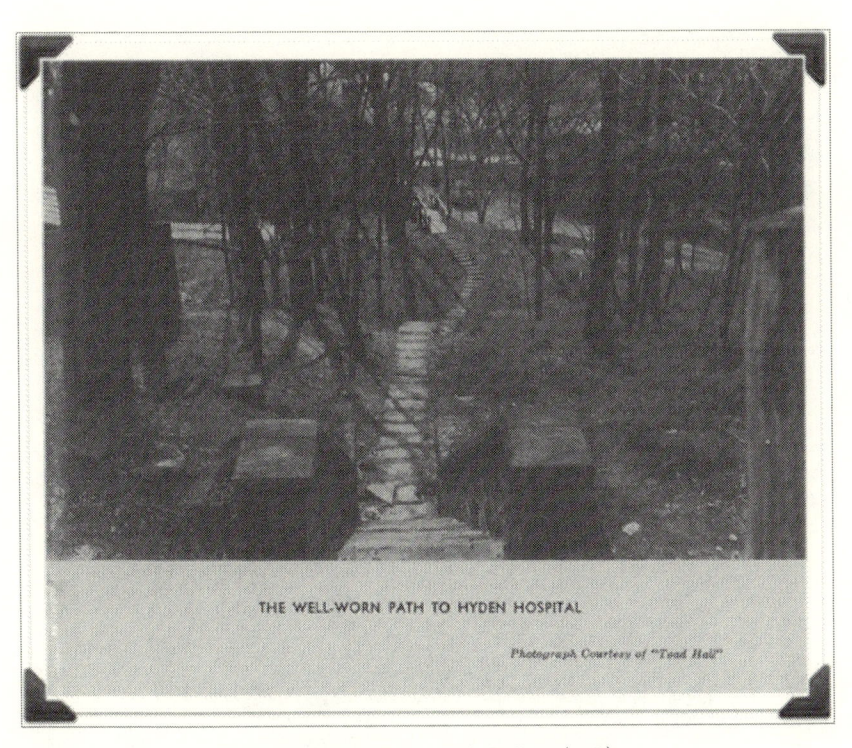

THE WELL-WORN PATH TO HYDEN HOSPITAL

Photograph Courtesy of "Toad Hall"

Spring 1974 FNS Quarterly Bulletin (14Q)

138

WEE STONE HOUSE
SOURCE: FNU ARCHIVES

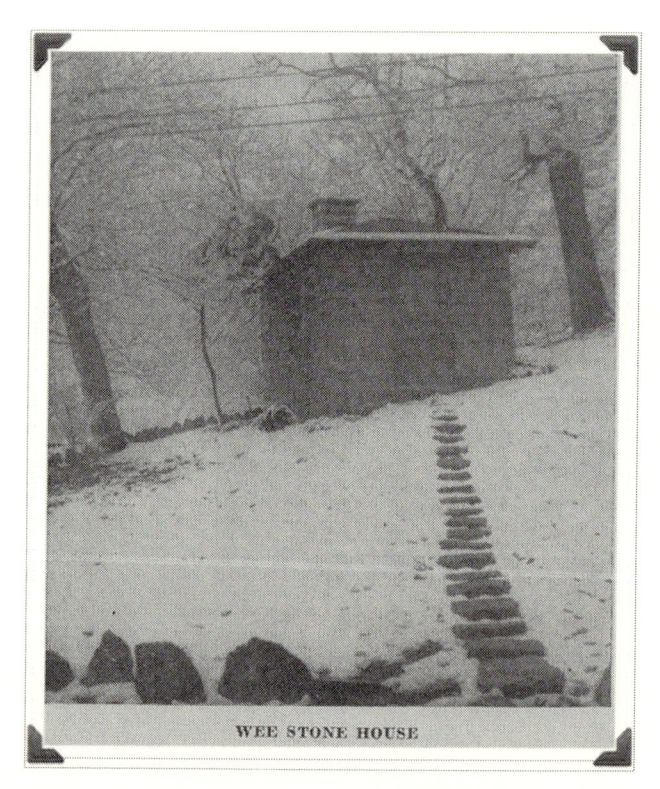

Winter 1943 FNS Quarterly Bulletin (14R)

139

THE UPPER SHELF
SOURCE: FNU ARCHIVES

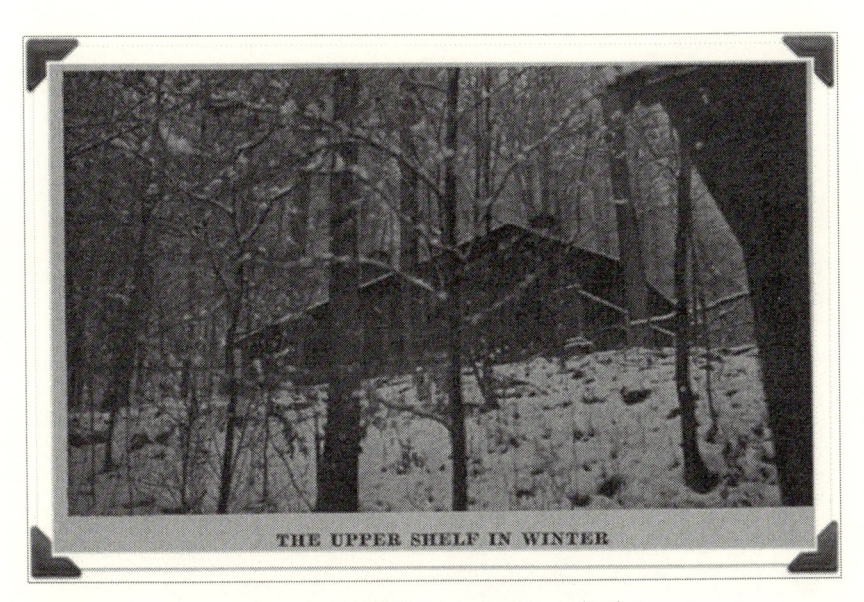

Autumn 1944 FNS Quarterly Bulletin (14S)

140

PARTY AT THE UPPER SHELF
SOURCE: FNU ARCHIVES

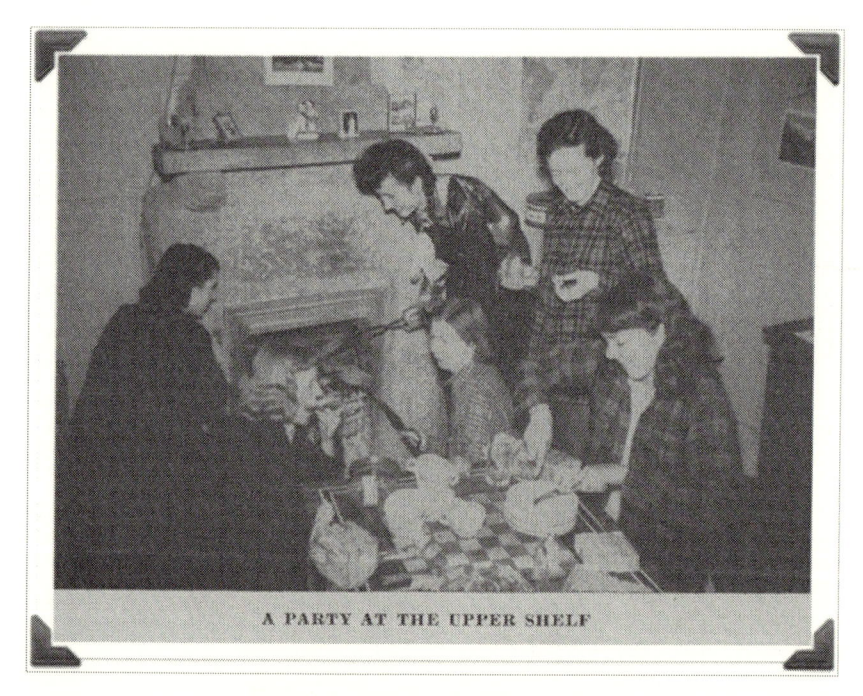

A PARTY AT THE UPPER SHELF

Autumn 1944 FNS Quarterly Bulletin (14T)

MARY FRANCES MORGAN
SOURCE: FNU ARCHIVES

WENDOVER CHRISTMAS PLAY

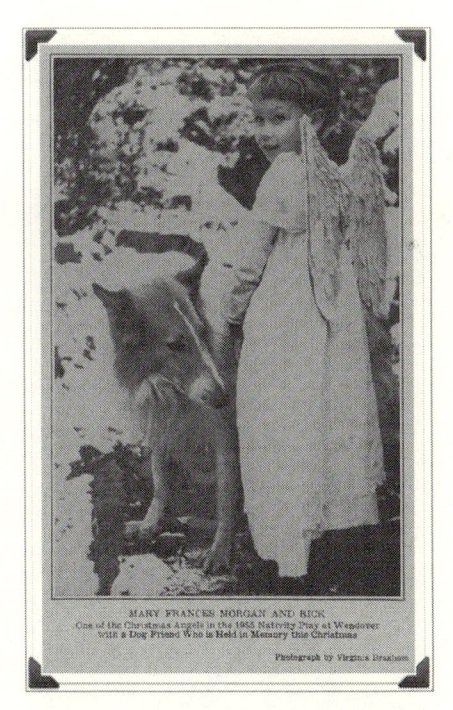

Autumn 1956 FNS Quarterly Bulletin (14U)

142

EARLY DAYS
SOURCE: FNU ARCHIVES

LIVING ROOM OF THE BIG HOUSE

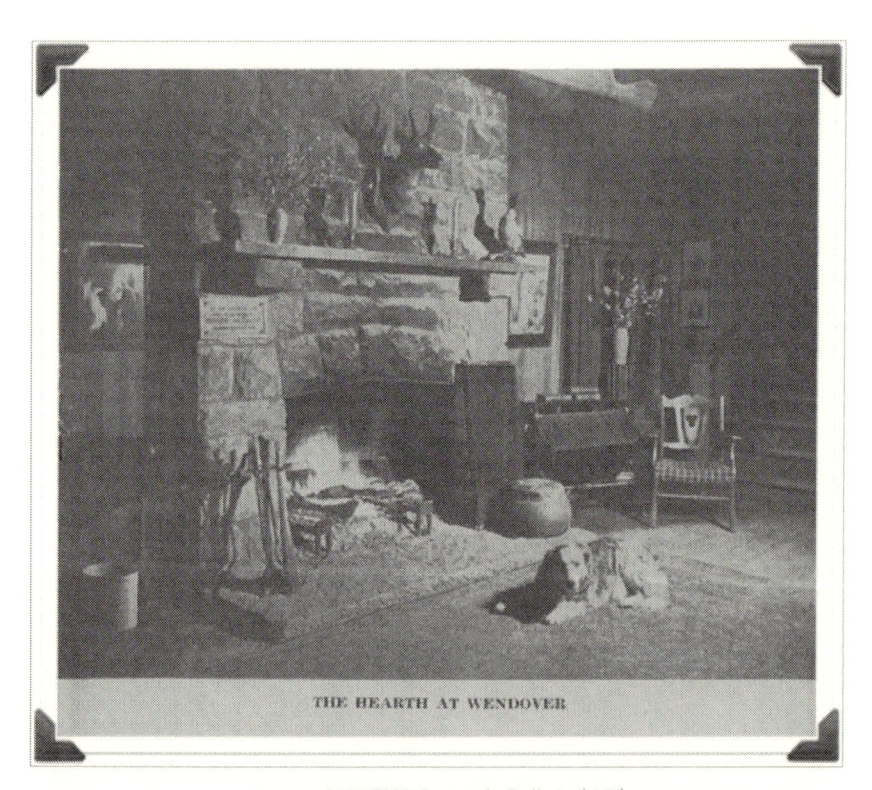

Autumn 1937 FNS Quarterly Bulletin (14V)

143
MOUNTAIN HOME VISIT
SOURCE: FNU ARCHIVES

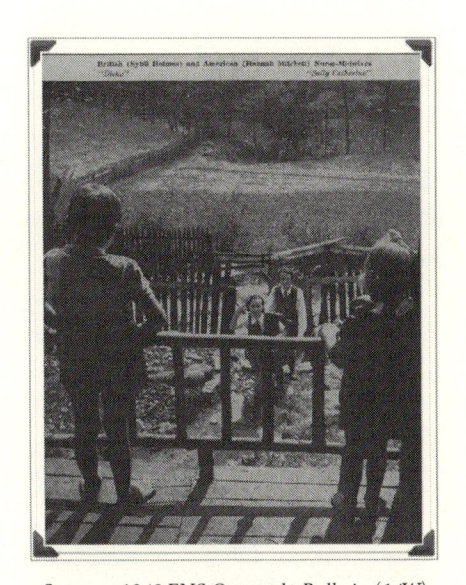

Summer 1940 FNS Quarterly Bulletin (14W)

144

KATE IRELAND
SOURCE: FNU ARCHIVES

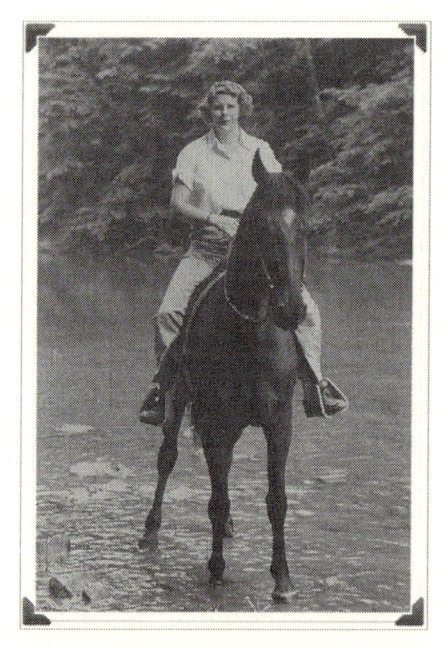

Winter 1986 FNS Quarterly Bulletin (14X)

145

MARY BRECKINRIDGE HOSPITAL
SOURCE: FNU ARCHIVES
PHOTO BY RUFUS FUGATE

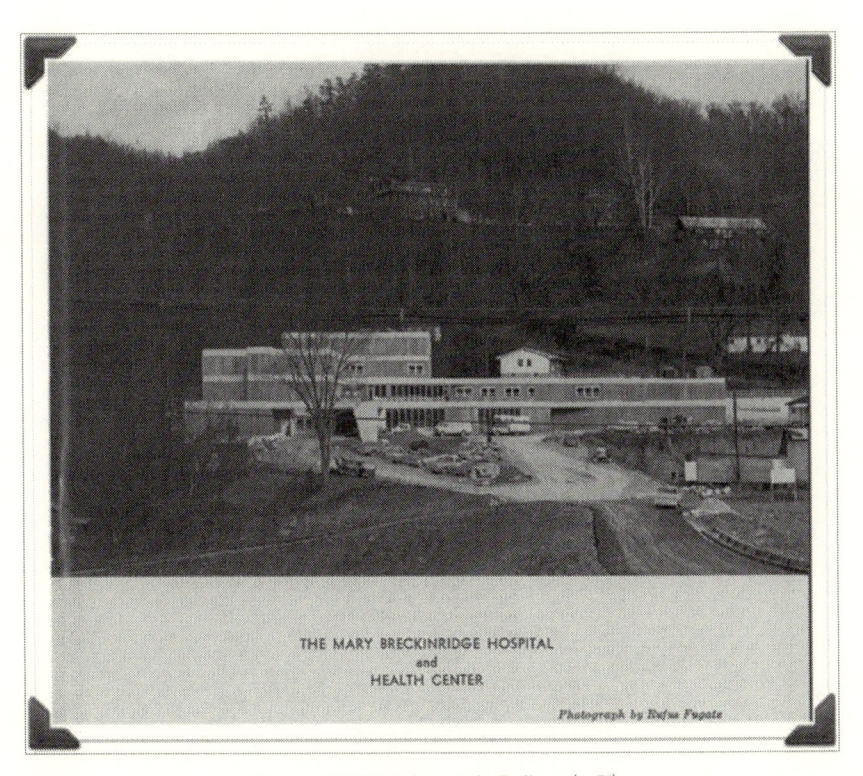

Winter 1975 FNS Quarterly Bulletin (14Y)

146

CORNERSTONE CONTENTS
SOURCE: FNU ARCHIVES

PHOTOS BY GABRIELLE BEASLEY

THE MARY BRECKINRIDGE HOSPITAL
Dedication Ceremony

CORNERSTONE CONTENTS

Helen E. Browne presents the contents of the cornerstone to Mrs. A. E. Cornett and Miss Betty Lester.

Gabrielle Beasley

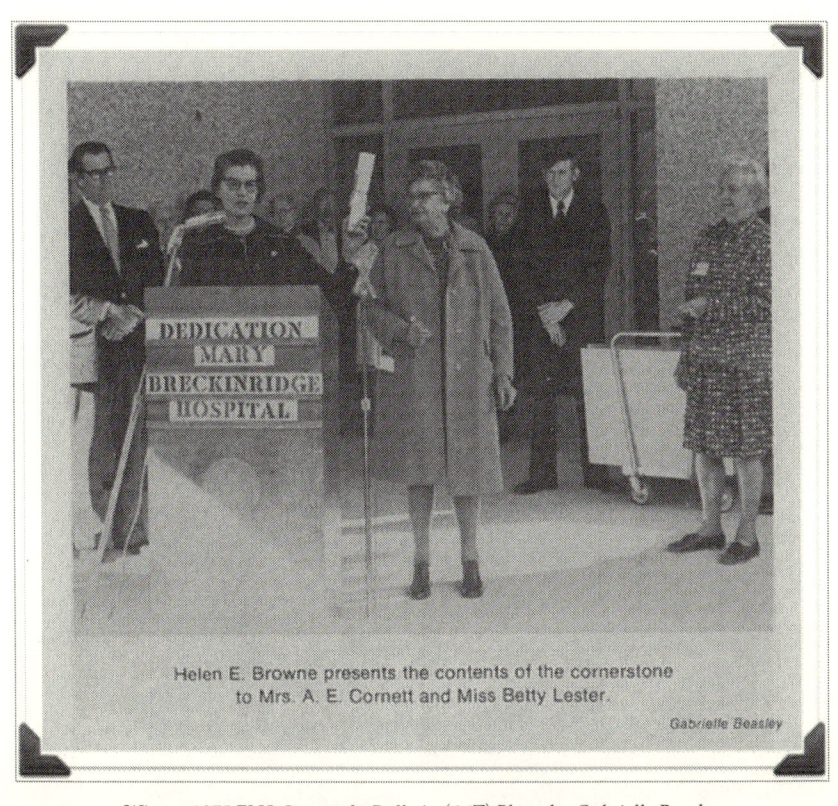

Winter 1975 FNS Quarterly Bulletin (14Z) Photo by Gabrielle Beasley

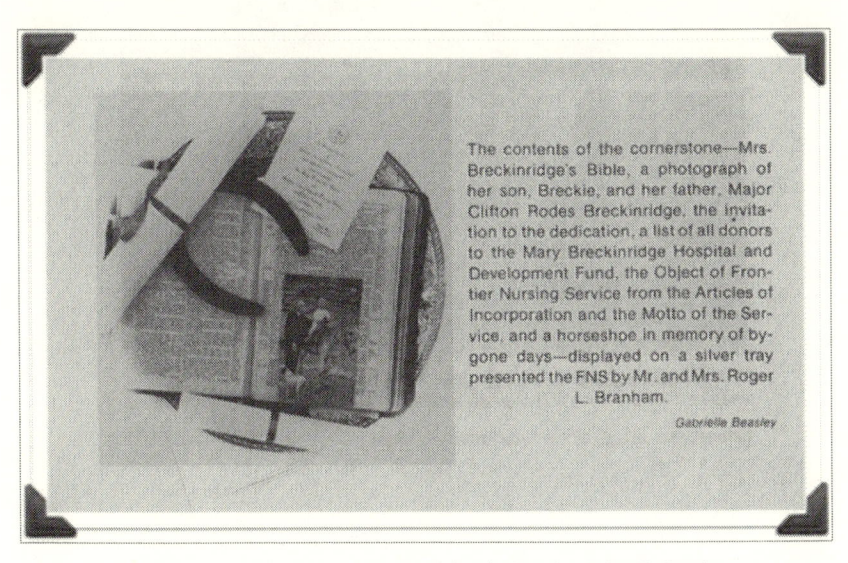

The contents of the cornerstone—Mrs. Breckinridge's Bible, a photograph of her son, Breckie, and her father, Major Clifton Rodes Breckinridge, the invitation to the dedication, a list of all donors to the Mary Breckinridge Hospital and Development Fund, the Object of Frontier Nursing Service from the Articles of Incorporation and the Motto of the Service, and a horseshoe in memory of bygone days—displayed on a silver tray presented the FNS by Mr. and Mrs. Roger L. Branham.

Gabrielle Beasley

Winter 1975 FNS Quarterly Bulletin (15A) Photo by Gabrielle Beasley

147

CHASTITY LYNN DEBORD
SOURCE: FNU ARCHIVES

FIRST BABY BORN IN THE NEW MARY BRECKINRIDGE HOSPITAL

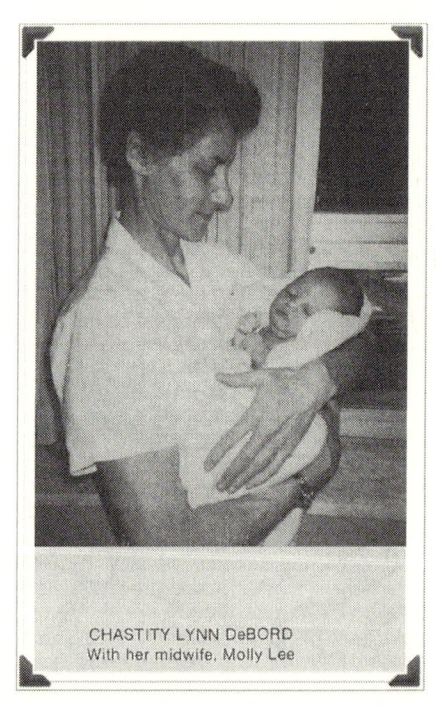

Winter 1975 FNS Quarterly Bulletin (15B)

148

SAYINGS OF OUR CHILDREN
SOURCE: FNU ARCHIVES
QUOTE BY TINA MCKINNEY

SAYINGS OF OUR CHILDREN

A four-year-old asked Granny to fix her favorite meal: "Chicken warts and Hockey beans".
Translation: Chicken livers and Shuckey beans.
—Contributed

Summer 1974 FNS Quarterly Bulletin (15C)

MY COUSIN'S response when she informed Sharon Koser that she'd had her most favorite meal—chicken warts and hockey beans. What she meant is that she'd eaten *chicken livers and shuckey beans.*

149

MOUNTAIN SCHOOLHOUSE
SOURCE: FNU ARCHIVES
ARTIST UNKNOWN

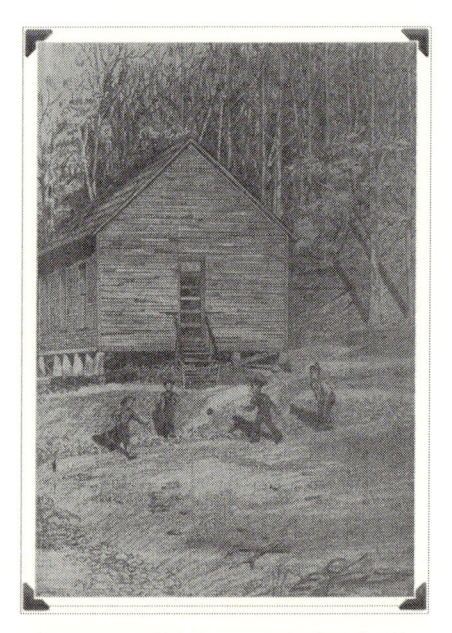

Spring 1953 FNS Quarterly Bulletin (15D)

150

GLORIA NAPIER
SOURCE: FNU ARCHIVES

LITTLEST ANGEL

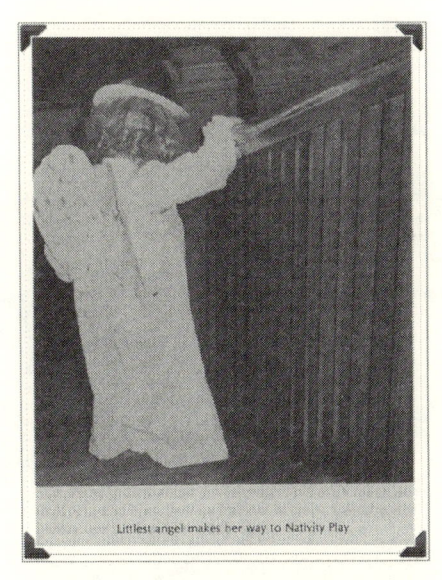

Autumn 1979 FNS Quarterly Bulletin (15E)

151

COAL COUNTRY GRASS
SOURCE: FNU ARCHIVES

LOCAL MUSICIANS DONATE PROCEEDS TO THE LESLIE COUNTY VOLUNTEER FIRE DEPARTMENT

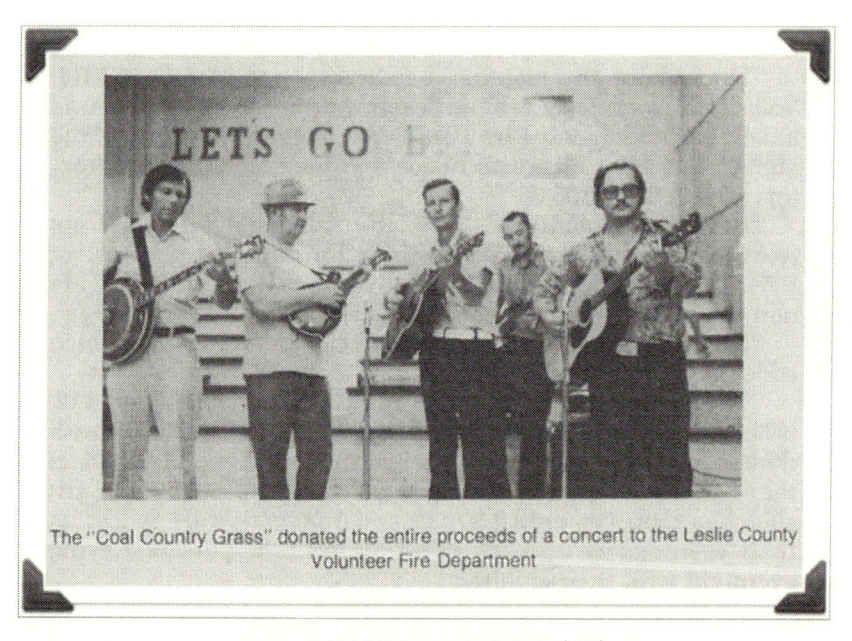

The "Coal Country Grass" donated the entire proceeds of a concert to the Leslie County Volunteer Fire Department

Spring 1978 FNS Quarterly Bulletin (15F)

152

NATIVITY PLAY
SOURCE: FNU ARCHIVES

AT WENDOVER GARDEN HOUSE

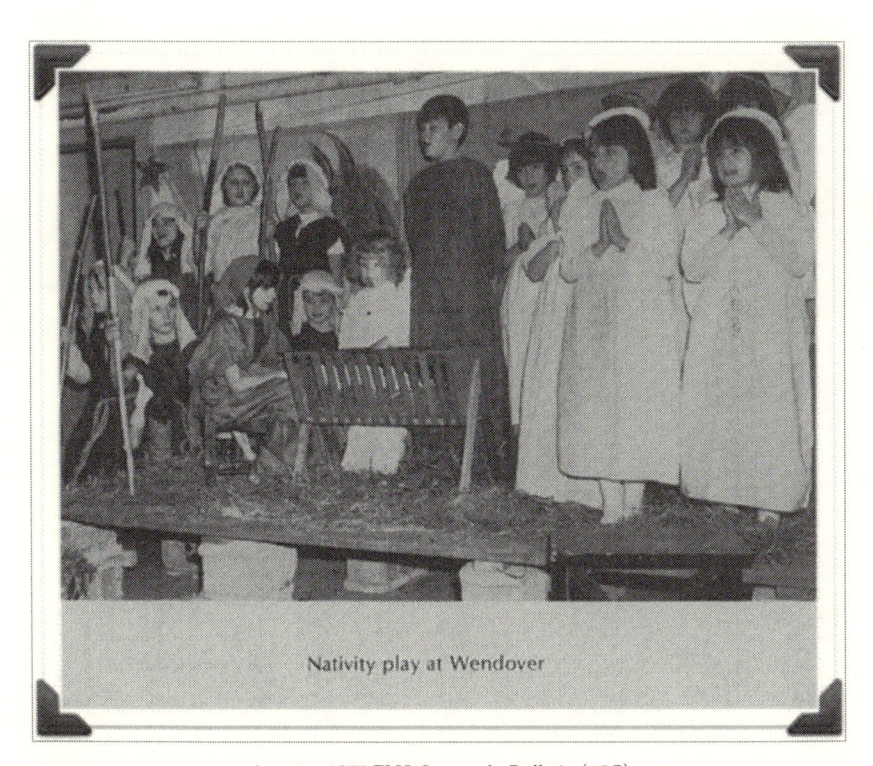

Autumn 1979 FNS Quarterly Bulletin (15G)

153

CHRISTMAS PLAY
SOURCE: FNU ARCHIVES
AT WENDOVER GARDEN HOUSE

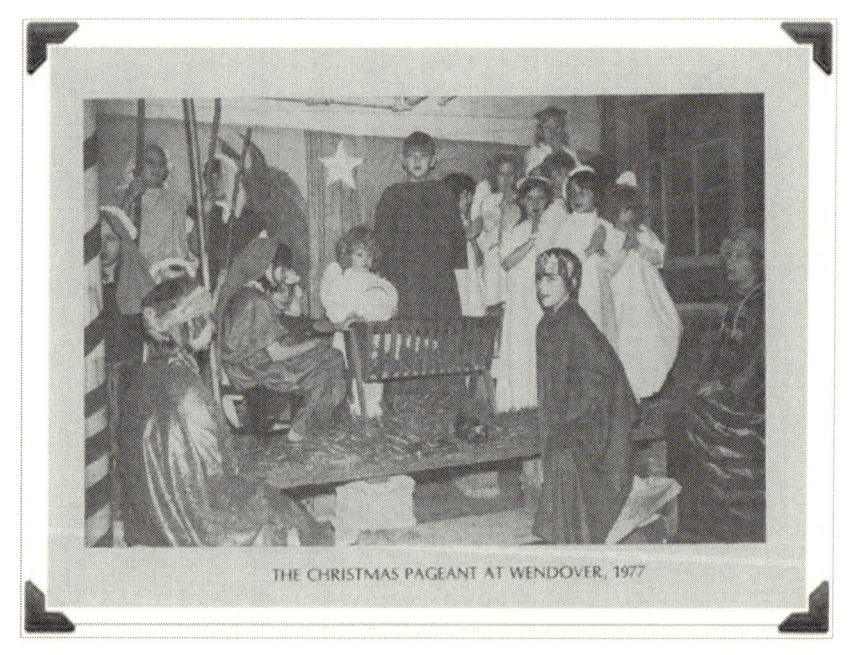

THE CHRISTMAS PAGEANT AT WENDOVER, 1977

Autumn 1977 FNS Quarterly Bulletin (15H)

154

GRETCHEN SHEPHERD
SOURCE: FNU ARCHIVES
CENTENNIAL PRINCESS

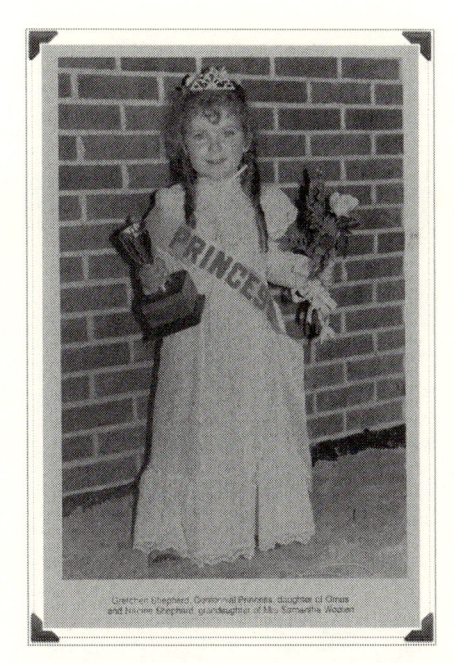

Summer 1978 FNS Quarterly Bulletin (15I)

155

BETTY LESTER

SOURCE: FNU ARCHIVES

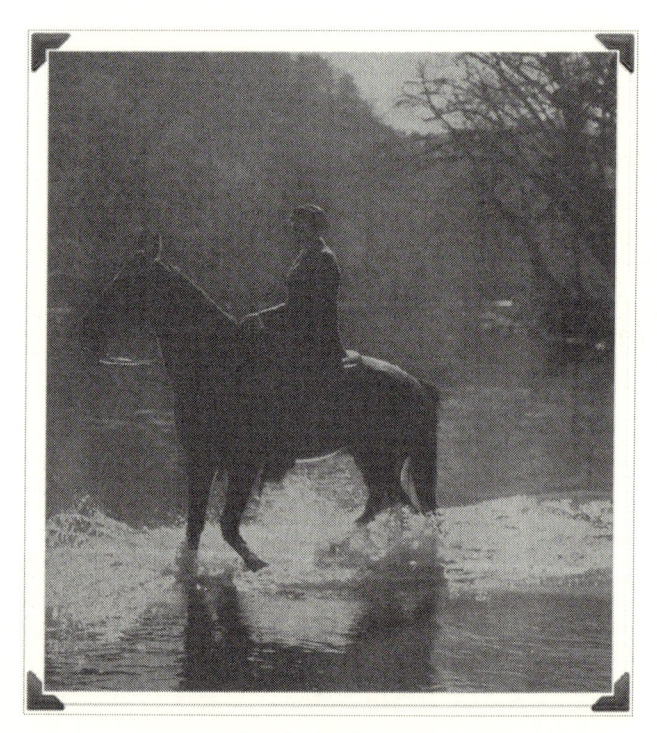

Spring 1934 FNS Quarterly Bulletin (15J)

156

CHRISTMAS NATIVITY PLAY
SOURCE: FNU ARCHIVES

RE-ENACTMENT BY LOCAL CHILDREN

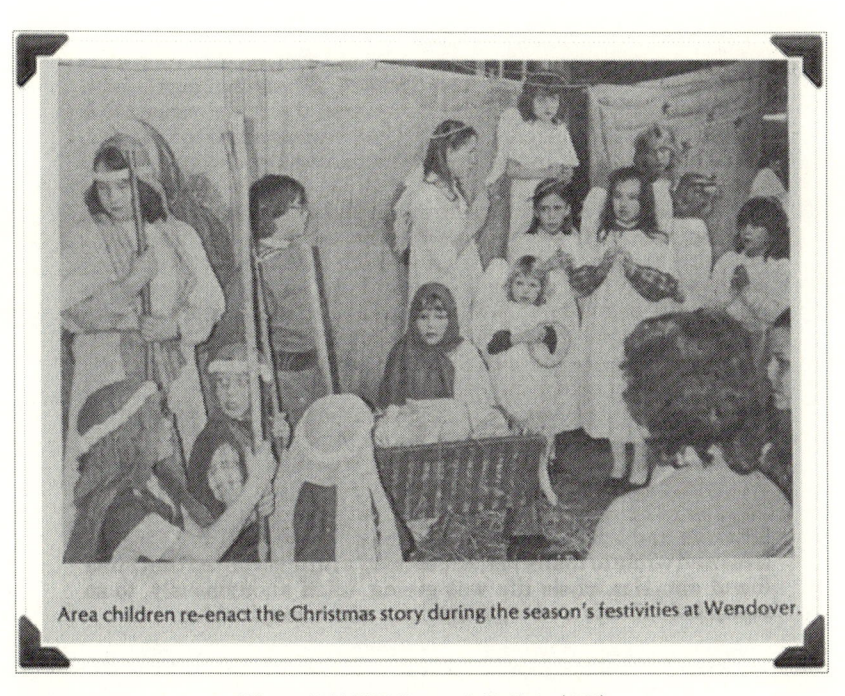

Area children re-enact the Christmas story during the season's festivities at Wendover.

Winter 1983 FNS Quarterly Bulletin (15K)

157

NATIVITY PAGEANT ANGELS
SOURCE: FNU ARCHIVES
WENDOVER

Autumn 1950 FNS Quarterly Bulletin (15L)

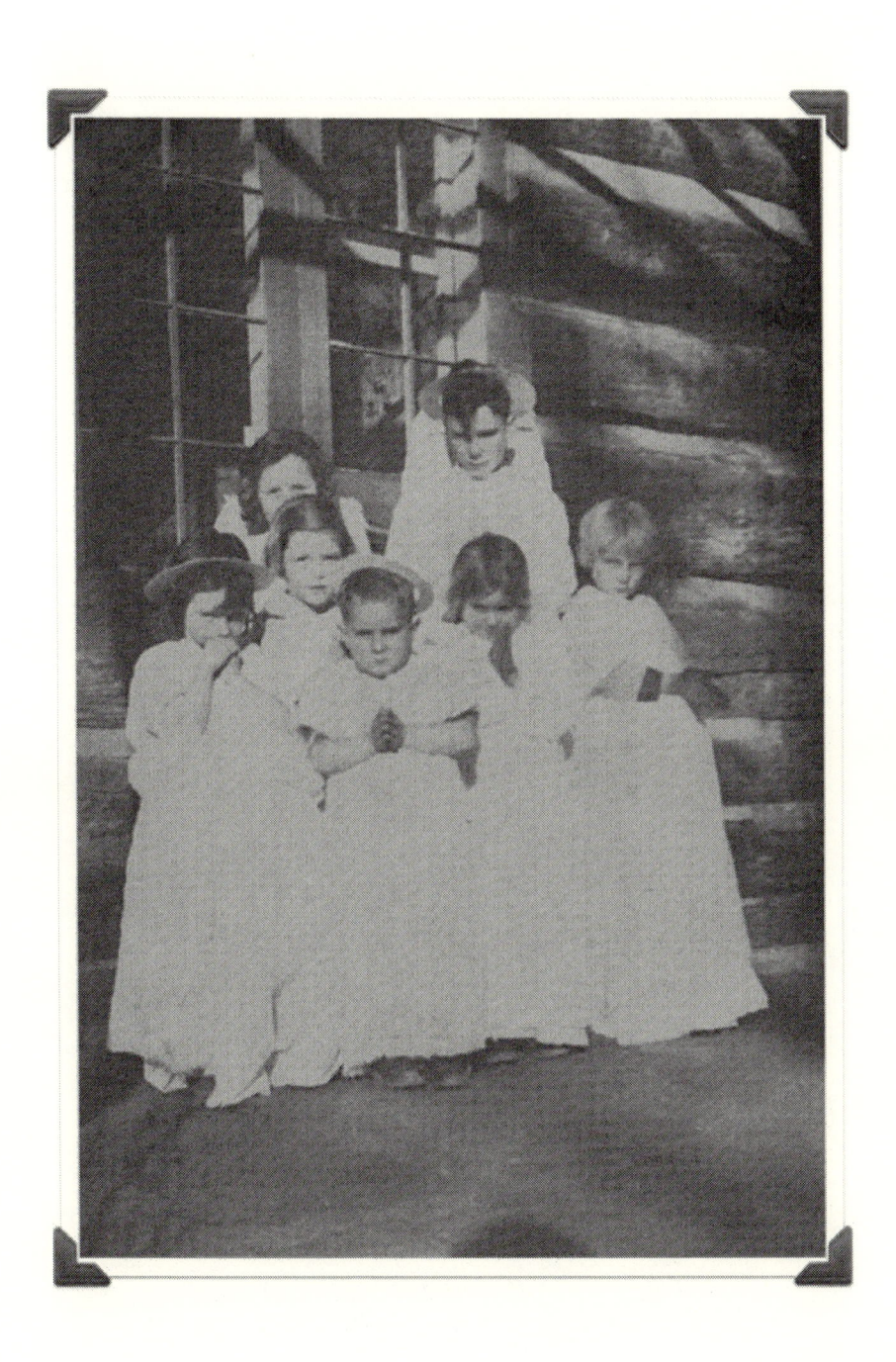

158

CHRISTMAS NATIVITY PAGEANT SHEPHERDS AND WISEMEN

SOURCE: FNU ARCHIVES

WENDOVER

AUTUMN 1950 QUARTERLY Bulletin (15M)

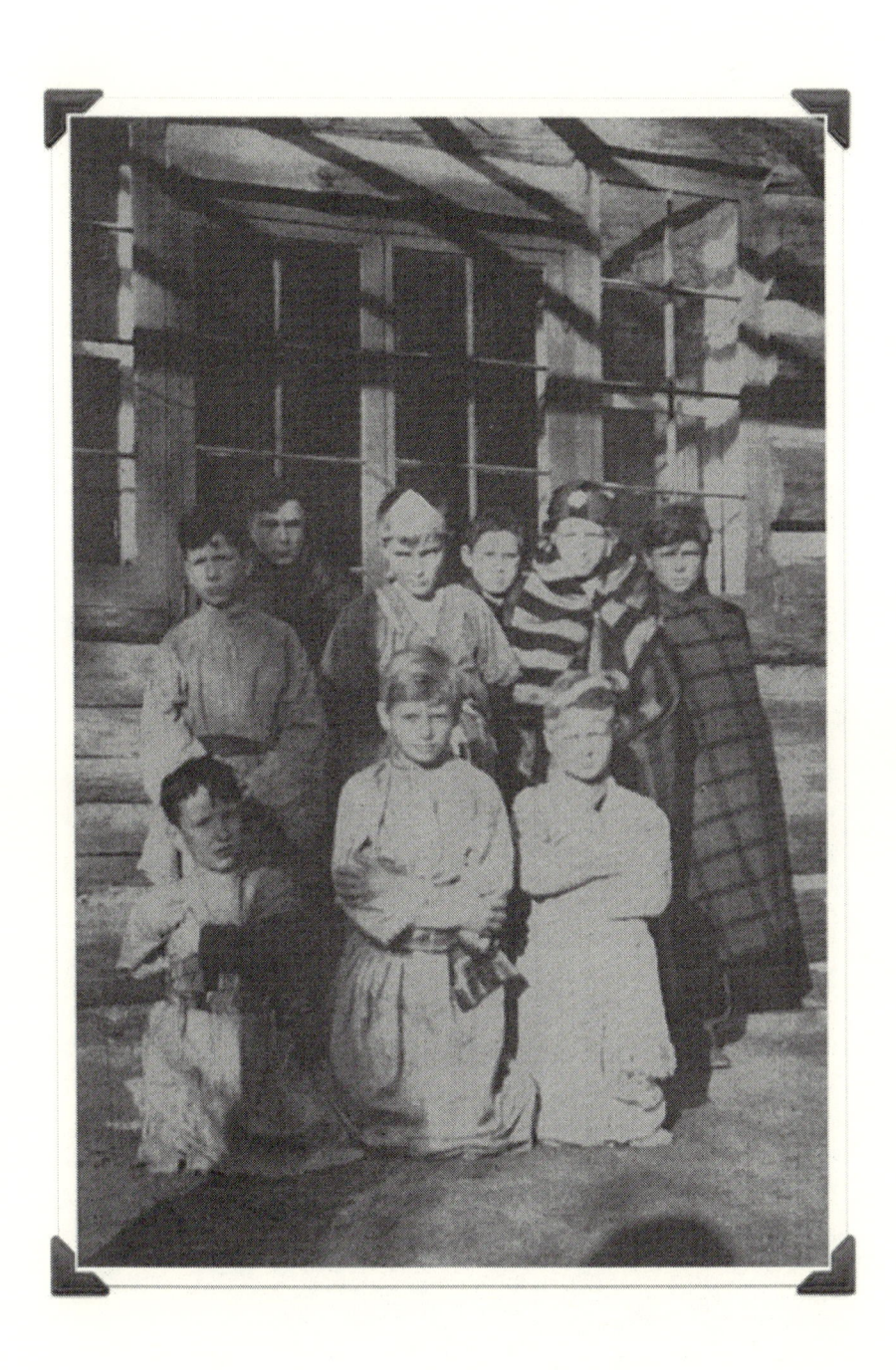

159

GRATITUDE

I BEGAN this book with a rather perplexing question:

"Could one dollar possibly change your life? How about something that was absolutely free?"

ZERO DOLLARS.

Do you think something that didn't cost a thing could possibly change your life? I know it changed mine. It changed mine; it changed the lives of the residents of Leslie County, and it changed healthcare as we know it in our little hometown of Hyden, Kentucky.

BUT HOW?

. . .

According to oral history, in 1925, Taylor Morgan gifted the Wendover property—the property where the Big House sits—to Mary Breckinridge. [F][G]

Nearly twenty years later, in 1941, the deed books record a property transaction for one dollar between Sally Morgan—widow of Taylor Morgan—and the Frontier Nursing Service. Sally Morgan's son, Pearl Morgan, and his wife, May, are also mentioned in this one dollar transaction. [F][G][E][13]

Deed book 42, page 403. (13)

Oral history suggests that this took place to show a legal transfer of property that had initially been a gift.

One little dollar.

I'm forever grateful to the Morgans because, had Mary Breckinridge settled in any other part of the county, I wouldn't have the same memories I have of FNS.

Had the Frontier Nursing Service not have been located on Wendover, right around the corner from the holler I grew up in, my FNS memories would have been quite different.

Mary Breckinridge was a gift to the citizens of our small town. In life, we all make our mark on this great big world, and I'm so thankful she chose our little corner of the world, in the hills of Eastern Kentucky, our Appalachian hometown, Hyden, Kentucky.

I've included the information on where to find the deed for the transaction. And in all the pages leading up to this one, I've explained in great detail what transpired after that transaction took place—the moment our legacy was set into motion...

~ *Amy Pennington Brudnicki*

160

ACKNOWLEDGEMENTS

I'd like to thank some very special people who have helped me along the way in getting this book ready for publication.

Without each of your contributions, this book would never have seen the light of day.

To **Cathy Eaves**, *I need to thank you for a phenomenal suggestion. You suggested that I use a picture of the stained glass window—from St. Christopher's Chapel—for a book cover.*

It was a wonderful suggestion, and one that inspired a truly special record of Leslie County history.

To **Michael Claussen**—*my favorite Wendover Historian—your assistance on this book has been extremely helpful and so very appreciated.*

Keep sharing your knowledge of Mary Breckinridge and the Frontier Nursing Service.

I never dreamed when I met you five years ago that a city boy from

Chicago could teach me a single thing about Mary Breckinridge. But, you schooled me six ways from Sunday on my own heritage. That's impressive.

I'D LIKE to thank my Mom, PEGGY LOVETT COVEY, for sharing some wonderful oral history with me and to my sister, KIM PENNINGTON HUFFMAN, for helping prompt ideas to expand on stories and photos.

Mom, thank you for taking the time to share your memories with us from Wendover and the old Hyden Hospital. Because of this, we have a better understanding of how things were all those years ago.

TO MY HUSBAND, WILLIAM BRUDNICKI, thank you for helping me with whatever I needed in the moment I needed it. Sometimes that was a listening ear, sometimes it was critical thinking, and sometimes it was giving suggestions that enriched some guided journal prompts.

You've heard so much about Mary Breckinridge, you probably feel like you're an FNS baby!

You're my favorite City Boy from Chicago, and I appreciate your willingness to revisit a Frontier you've never known.

TO ELBERT ESTEP, I want to say thank you. Thank you for taking such a striking photo of St. Christopher's Chapel and that gorgeous stained glass window, and thank you for allowing me to include it in this book.

You have a God given talent for photography, and I'm forever grateful that you share that with the world.

TO AUDREY MAGGARD CLOWERS, thanks for the help with the beautiful quote and in keeping me straight on some details.

. . .

AMY PENNINGTON BRUDNICKI

To **Patricia McKinney**, I'd like to thank you for the pictures that you allowed me to use from the Wendover Christmas Plays. What a wonderful time in our lives.

To **Audrey Maggard**, **Mary Collins**, **Leona Begley**, **Helen Maggard**, and **Patricia McKinney**, thank you for sharing stories over the years about Mary Breckinridge, Wendover, and FNS.

To **Angela Bailey**, thank you for all your help with getting the permission to use these vintage FNS pictures and quarterly bulletin pictures in this book. I appreciate your willingness to work with me, and I appreciate you being so kind no matter how many email exchanges we had.

To **Debbie Farley**, thank you for the help with resources.

To **Wendy Collett**, thank you for taking a picture of me during my book signing at The Big House. It captured a moment in time that I'd otherwise be without. Also, thank you for allowing me to include it in my book.

To **Melody Claussen**, thank you for allowing me to include your photo. We had such a great day that day.

To **Alma Browning**, thank you so much for the last minute request. You came through for me in a pinch, and I appreciate you dearly!

. . .

REMEMBERING THE FRONTIER

To **Carla Cantagallo** and **Colleen Barrett** with the **University of Kentucky Libraries' Special Collection's Research Center**, I want to say thank you. You ladies helped me find direction when I was first getting started with this book, and I am forever grateful for your assistance.

To **Brittney Kinison**, thank you for all your help with getting the permission to use these FNS pictures in this book. I appreciate your willingness to work with me.

To **Billie Anne Gebb**, thank you for helping me obtain the permission to use the FNS Quarterly Bulletins in my book.

To **Jennifer Asher** with the **Leslie County PVA office**, thank you for your assistance in obtaining the deed I was looking for. You've been so helpful to me and always incredibly gracious. I appreciate you, girl!

To **Grace Napier**, thank you for the idea to include the deed in my book. In the end, the picture quality wasn't clear enough to include it. Still yet, it was a phenomenal idea.

The Morgan family is directly responsible for Mary Breckinridge choosing the property she did on Wendover, and for that, I am forever grateful to them.

To **Onzie Sizemore** and the **Leslie County Court Clerk's Office**, thank you for the help with the deed.

. . .

To **Agnes Melton**, *thank you for reminiscing with me and sharing your FNS history. It was a wonderful journey back in time.*

When we were discussing Wendover, you referred to the Christmas plays as, "Pageants." I had seen them referred to as "Pageants" in the Quarterly Bulletins. It occurred to me that each generation called them something different. I imagine that was the result of the program coordinator. I'm sure we called it whatever they called it.

But, after our conversation, I expanded on what I'd originally written. Because of our conversation, I told a richer story. Thank you for the inspiration.

To **Audrey Morgan Maggard**, *thank you for telling me stories about Mary Breckinridge.*

It was so special to see her through the eyes of a child, and because you shared your story with me, I was able to do that.

To **Carolyn Estep Myers**, *thank you for sharing your FNS memories with me.*

To **Raegan Napier Caldwell** *and* **Eileen Morgan**, *thank you for helping me track down a very special photo.*

To **Katharyne Shelton**, *thank you for brainstorming with me.*

To **Frontier Nursing University**, *I appreciate you allowing me to use these pictures in my book.*

. . .

To ALL the Leslie County historians—past and present—I want to say thank you. Because you took the time to record a memory, to share a story, to note a moment in time, my generation and future generations have a better understanding of our little hometown that we hold so dear.

To be a historian, you simply need to be willing to share what you know and what you've experienced, and I'm so very thankful that you have.

To EVERYONE who takes the time to share your FNS memories with loved ones, I want to say thank you. The information you're providing is preserving history for future generations.

I appreciate you all,

~ Amy

THIS MAY BE UNCONVENTIONAL, but it's my book, and I'm doing it my way. I want to say thank you to myself. Someday, when my mind gets tired, I'll appreciate having all these facts in one spot about the town that built me.

Sometimes, the person we record memories for is ourselves.

IT's my mission to assure that the Frontier is never forgotten . . .

~Amy Pennington Brudnicki

REFERENCES

Oral History

A. Michael Claussen
　B. Peggy Lovett Covey
　C. Oral History passed down from generation to generation—so much so, we have no idea where it originated. This reference includes history from family members: Orlena Maggard, Hazel Lovett, Audrey Maggard, Mary Collins, Helen Maggard, Leona Begley, and Patricia McKinney.
　D. Agnes Melton
　E. Grace Napier
　F. Amy Maggard Sizemore
　G. Audrey Morgan Maggard

162

REFERENCES

SOURCES

1. *Business Insider 2018, accessed September 11, 2020,<www.businessinsider.com/how-much-does-it-cost-to-have-a-baby-2018-4>*

2. *Historic FNS photos, FNU*

3. *FNS Quarterly Bulletins, FNU*

- *3A Frontier Nursing Service Quarterly Bulletin, Vol. 40, No. 4, Spring 1965, front cover, pages 4, 5.*
- *3B The Quarterly Bulletin of The Kentucky Committee for Mothers and Babies, Inc., Vol. III, No. 3, November 1927, page 3.*
- *3C The Quarterly Bulletin of The Frontier Nursing Service, Inc., Vol. IV, No. 2, September 1928, pages 1-3.*

(3Da)The Quarterly Bulletin of The Frontier Nursing Service, Inc., Vol. 32, No. 2, Autumn 1956, page 57.

(3Db) *Frontier Nursing Service Quarterly Bulletin, Vol. 36, No. 2, Autumn 1960, inside cover.*
(3Dc) *Frontier Nursing Service Quarterly Bulletin, Vol. 38, No. 2, Autumn 1962, inside cover.*
(3Dd) *Frontier Nursing Service Quarterly Bulletin, Vol. 55, No. 2, Autumn 1979, inside cover.*

- *3E Frontier Nursing Service Quarterly Bulletin, Vol. 40, No. 4, Spring 1965, page 4.*
- *3F The Quarterly Bulletin of The Frontier Nursing Service, Inc., Vol. 25, No. 4, Spring 1950, pages 30, 31.*
- *3G Frontier Nursing Service Quarterly Bulletin, Vol. 37, No. 2, Autumn 1961, pages 3-10.*
- *3H*
- *The Quarterly Bulletin of The Frontier Nursing Service, Inc., Vol. 18, No. 2, Autumn 1942, pages 13-17.*
- *The Quarterly Bulletin of The Frontier Nursing Service, Inc., Vol. XVII, No. 3, Winter 1942, pages 3-15.*
- *3I The Quarterly Bulletin of The Frontier Nursing Service, Inc., Vol. 20, No. 2, Autumn 1944, pages 25-28.*
- *3Ja Frontier Nursing Service Quarterly Bulletin, Vol. 33, No. 3, Winter 1958, page 5.*
- *3Jb Frontier Nursing Service Quarterly Bulletin, Vol. 33, No. 3, Winter 1958, page 6.*
- *3K The Quarterly Bulletin of The Frontier Nursing Service, Inc., Vol. 18, No. 3, Winter 1943, page 81, photo.*
- *3L Frontier Nursing Service Quarterly Bulletin, Vol. 35, No. 4, Spring 1960, page 3.*
- *3M Frontier Nursing Service Quarterly Bulletin, Vol. 35, No. 3, Winter 1960, page 36.*
- *3N Frontier Nursing Service Quarterly Bulletin, Vol. 35, No. 4, Spring 1960, page 5.*
- *3O Frontier Nursing Service Quarterly Bulletin, Vol. 36, No. 3, Winter 1961, page 8.*
- *3P Frontier Nursing Service Quarterly Bulletin, Vol. 52, No. 2, Autumn 1976, pages 5-6.*

- 3Q *Frontier Nursing Service Quarterly Bulletin, Vol. 50, No. 3, Winter 1975, page 5.*
- 3R *Frontier Nursing Service Quarterly Bulletin, Vol. 50, No. 2, Autumn 1974, page 3.*
- 3S *Frontier Nursing Service Quarterly Bulletin, Vol. 46, No. 2, Autumn 1970, page 15.*
- 3T *Frontier Nursing Service Quarterly Bulletin, Vol. 36, No. 3, Winter 1961, inside cover.*
- 3U *The Quarterly Bulletin of The Frontier Nursing Service, Inc., Vol. 24, No. 3, Winter 1949, page 28.*
- 3V *The Quarterly Bulletin of The Frontier Nursing Service, Inc., Vol. 24, No. 3, Winter 1949, page 29.*
- 3W *Frontier Nursing Service Quarterly Bulletin, Vol. 50, No. 3, Winter 1975, page 6.*
- 3X *Frontier Nursing Service Quarterly Bulletin, Vol. VI, No. 4, Spring 1931, Front Cover.*

4. *Wide Neighborhoods* by Mary Breckinridge, page 121

5. *Wikipedia 2020, accessed September 11, 2020,*

<https://en.wikipedia.org/wiki/Mary_Carson_Breckinridge>

6. *National Museum of American History: Midwives on Horseback: Saddlebags and Science by Dr. Laura Ettinger, March 25, 2015* <https://americanhistory.si.edu/blog/midwives-horseback-saddlebags-and-science>

7. *Scholar Works Morehead State University, Leslie County - Post Offices & Places Names, The Post Offices of Leslie County, May 27, 1978, accessed September 2, 2020.* <https://scholarworks.moreheadstate.edu/cgi/viewcontent.cgi?article=1243&context=kentucky_county_histories>

8. *Society of Architectural Historians,*

<"Wendover", [Hyden, Kentucky], SAH Archipedia, eds. Gabrielle Esperdy and Karen Kingsley, Charlottesville: UVaP, 2012—, http://sah-archipedia.org/buildings/KY-01-131-0093. Last accessed, September 12, 2020.

9. *A great site for looking up old FNS Quarterly Bulletins,* <exploreuk.uky.edu>.

10. *Wikipedia 2019, accessed September 16, 2020,*

<https://en.wikipedia.org/wiki/Riderless_horse>

11. TopScholar 1993, *Made to Fit a Woman: Riding Uniforms of the Frontier Nursing Service* by Donna C. Parker, accessed September 17, 2020, <https://digitalcommons.wku.edu/dlsc_fac_pub/20/>

12. University of Kentucky Uknowledge, *The Frontier Nursing Service Oral History Project: An Annotated Guide*, Susan E. Allen, Accessed October 14, 2020, https://uknowledge.uky.edu/cgi/viewcontent.cgi?article=1000&context=libraries_papers, page 26.

13. Leslie County PVA & Leslie County Court Clerk Deed from Sally Morgan to the Frontier Nursing Service. Deed book 42, page 403.

14. FNS Quarterly Bulletins, Cropped for Photos:

14A The Kentucky Committee for Mothers and Babies Quarterly Bulletin, Vol. I, No. 1, June 1925, Front Cover.

14B The Quarterly Bulletin of The Frontier Nursing Service, Inc., Vol. VII, No. 1, Summer 1931, Front Cover.

14C The Quarterly Bulletin of The Frontier Nursing Service, Inc., Vol. V, No. 1, June 1929, Front Cover.

14D Frontier Nursing Service Quarterly Bulletin, Vol. 36, No. 1, Summer 1960, page 17.

14E Frontier Nursing Service Quarterly Bulletin, Vol. 36, No. 2, Autumn 1960, page 5.

14F Frontier Nursing Service Quarterly Bulletin, Vol. 58, No. 2, Autumn 1982, Front Cover.

14G Frontier Nursing Service Quarterly Bulletin, Vol. 51, No. 2, Autumn 1975, page 5.

14H Frontier Nursing Service Quarterly Bulletin, Vol. 36, No. 2, Autumn 1960, inside front cover.

14I The Quarterly Bulletin of The Frontier Nursing Service, Inc., Vol. VI, No. 4, Spring 1931, Front Cover.

14J The Quarterly Bulletin of The Frontier Nursing Service, Inc., Vol. VI, No. 4, Spring 1931, Front Cover.

14K Frontier Nursing Service Quarterly Bulletin, Vol. 35, No. 4, Spring 1960, inside back cover.

14L Frontier Nursing Service Quarterly Bulletin, Vol. 52, No. 2, Autumn 1976, inside back cover.

14M Frontier Nursing Service Quarterly Bulletin, Vol. 52, No. 2, Autumn 1976, inside back cover.

14N The Quarterly Bulletin of The Frontier Nursing Service, Inc., Vol. VI, No. 3, Winter 1931, Front Cover.

14O Frontier Nursing Service Quarterly Bulletin, Vol. 50, No. 1, Summer 1974, Front Cover.

14P The Quarterly Bulletin of The Frontier Nursing Service, Inc., Vol. 30, No. 2, Autumn 1954, Front Cover.

14Q Frontier Nursing Service Quarterly Bulletin, Vol. 49, No. 4, Spring 1974, Front Cover.

14R The Quarterly Bulletin of The Frontier Nursing Service, Inc., Vol. 18, No. 3, Winter 1943, inside back cover.

14S The Quarterly Bulletin of The Frontier Nursing Service, Inc., Vol. 20, No. 2, Autumn 1944, page 25.

14T The Quarterly Bulletin of The Frontier Nursing Service, Inc., Vol. 20, No. 2, Autumn 1944, Page 26.

14U The Quarterly Bulletin of The Frontier Nursing Service, Inc., Vol. 32, No. 2, Autumn 1956, inside back cover.

14V The Quarterly Bulletin of The Frontier Nursing Service, Inc., Vol. XIII, No. 2, Autumn 1937, Front Cover.

14W The Quarterly Bulletin of The Frontier Nursing Service, Inc., Vol. XVI, No. 1, Summer 1940, Front Cover.

14X Frontier Nursing Service Quarterly Bulletin, Vol. 61, No. 3, Winter 1986, Front Cover.

14Y Frontier Nursing Service Quarterly Bulletin, Vol. 50, No. 3, Winter 1975, Front Cover.

14Z Frontier Nursing Service Quarterly Bulletin, Vol. 50, No. 3, Winter 1975, page 6.

15. *FNS Quarterly Bulletins, Cropped for Photos:*

15A Frontier Nursing Service Quarterly Bulletin, Vol. 50, No. 3, Winter 1975, page 6.

15B Frontier Nursing Service Quarterly Bulletin, Vol. 50, No. 3, Winter 1975, page 24.

15C Frontier Nursing Service Quarterly Bulletin, Vol. 50, No. 1, Summer 1974, page 44.

15D The Quarterly Bulletin of The Frontier Nursing Service, Inc., Vol. 28, No. 4, Spring 1953, page 33.

15E Frontier Nursing Service Quarterly Bulletin, Vol. 55, No. 2, Autumn 1979, page 43.

15F Frontier Nursing Service Quarterly Bulletin, Vol. 53, No. 4, Spring 1978, page 35.

15G Frontier Nursing Service Quarterly Bulletin, Vol. 55, No. 2, Autumn 1979, inside cover.

15H Frontier Nursing Service Quarterly Bulletin, Vol. 53, No. 2, Autumn 1977, inside back cover.

15I Frontier Nursing Service Quarterly Bulletin, Vol. 54, No. 1, Summer 1978, page 73.

15J The Quarterly Bulletin of The Frontier Nursing Service, Inc., Vol. IX, No. 4, Spring 1934, Front Cover.

15K Frontier Nursing Service Quarterly Bulletin, Vol. 58, No. 3, Winter 1983, page 17.

AMY PENNINGTON BRUDNICKI

15L The Quarterly Bulletin of The Frontier Nursing Service, Inc., Vol. 26, No. 2, Autumn 1950, inside back cover.

15M The Quarterly Bulletin of The Frontier Nursing Service, Inc., Vol. 26, No. 2, Autumn 1950, inside back cover.

16. The J. Paul Getty Museum, Getty.edu, Saint Christopher carrying the Christ child, accessed November, 04, 2020 http://www.getty.edu/art/collection/objects/103432/spitz-master-saint-christopher-carrying-the-christ-child-french-about-1420/

+ *Special Note: At time of publication, the fate of The Wendover Bed & Breakfast is unknown.*

ABOUT THE AUTHOR

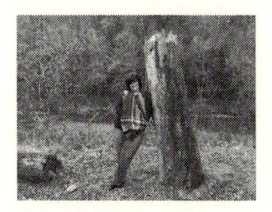

Amy Pennington Brudnicki was born and raised in Hyden, a quaint town in southeastern Kentucky. At an early age, she penned clandestine paranormal mysteries—nothing more than a page in length—and always quickly discarded. As a forlorn teen, she began to write poetry. Her collection was stored in a ratty old notebook and tucked away out of sight.

Throughout her life, she wrote tales that would evoke laughter in anyone who read them. This was all before the age of the Internet. Shortly after high school, Amy's home was destroyed by fire. She and her family lost everything they had, stories and poems included.

Thinking that writing was nothing more than a hobby, she laid her pen aside and focused on her education and starting a family. Years later, her old soul caught up with her as she felt that familiar pull once more. She has since written newspaper articles, a novel, a collection of short stories, and guided journals.

Her purpose in sharing this with you is to urge you not to give up on your dreams. She'd tell you that it's never too late to dream a new dream, just as it's never too late to explore one previously set aside . . .

facebook.com/amybru

ALSO BY AMY PENNINGTON BRUDNICKI

Echoes of the Past: My Dirt Road Diary

Memoirs, a guided journal by Old Soul Publications

My Life Reflections, a guided journal by Old Soul Publications

Old Soul Publications is my pen name when I publish journals.

Made in the USA
Coppell, TX
27 January 2023